Ignite *Your* Light

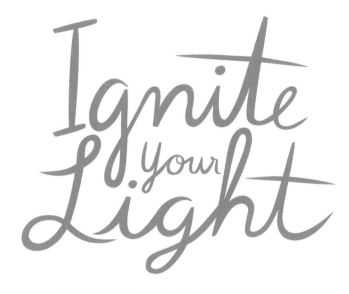

A SUNRISE-*to*-MOONLIGHT GUIDE
to FEELING JOYFUL, RESILIENT,
and LIT *from* WITHIN

JOLENE HART, CHC

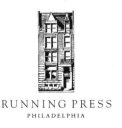

Running Press
PHILADELPHIA

Running Press
Hachette Book Group
1290 Avenue of the Americas, New York, NY 10104
www.runningpress.com
@Running_Press

Printed in China
First Trade Paperback Edition: June 2021

Published by Running Press, an imprint of Perseus Books, LLC, a subsidiary of Hachette Book Group, Inc. The Running Press name and logo is a trademark of the Hachette Book Group.

The Hachette Speakers Bureau provides a wide range of authors for speaking events. To find out more, go to www.hachettespeakersbureau.com or call (866) 376-6591.

The publisher is not responsible for websites (or their content) that are not owned by the publisher.

Photographs copyright © 2020 by Jolene Hart
Print book cover and interior design by Susan Van Horn.

Library of Congress Control Number: 2019951769

ISBNs: 978-0-7624-7467-7 (paperback), 978-0-7624-9614-3 (hardcover), 978-0-7624-9616-7 (ebook)

1010

11   10   9   8   7   6   5   4   3   2

For anyone who is lost in the dark—

may your light illuminate the path to a place of

beauty, resilience, and joy.

CONTENTS

Introduction 1

PART 1: THE ENERGY OF YOU AND ME 17

CHAPTER 1: **Be the Light You Want to See** 19

Define Your Energy Quiz 43

PART 2: YOUR ENERGETIC DAY 47

Introduction 48

CHAPTER 2: **Sunrise** 55

Sunrise Energy Influencers 60

Morning Messaging: The Energy of Your Mindset 61

Get Physical: The Energy of Movement 70

Well Begun: The Energy of Preparation 77

Recipes to Nourish Your Sunrise Energy 85

Sunday Morning Ginger-Apple Fritters with Raw Honey Glaze 86

Vacation Vibes Avocado Smoothie Bowl 89

Grounding Sunrise Omelet 90

Green Beauty Broth 92

Sesame Glow Bars 95

Spring Garden Galette 96

CHAPTER 3: **Daylight** 99

Daylight Energy Influencers 105

In the Flow: The Energy of Work and Creativity 105

Come Together: The Energy of Relationships and Connection 116

Your Anchor for Calm: The Energy of Breath 127

Recipes to Nourish Your Daylight Energy 135

Gingersnap Cashews 136

Coconut-Raspberry Love Bites 139

Fueled & Focused Salad with Superfood Sunflower Dressing 140

Jasmine Cacao Brain-Boosting Tonic 142

No-Time Niçoise Salad 145

Sunny Day Seed Crackers 146

CHAPTER 4: Sunset 149

Sunset Energy Influencers 153

Wild and Free: The Energy of Play and Laughter. 154

The Light Around You: The Energy of Interior Spaces 162

Good Vibrations: The Energy of Sound and Music 171

Recipes to Nourish Your Sunset Energy 177

    Sunset Chill Cocktail. 178

    Cashew Jalapeño Beans and Greens Bowl 181

    Miso Lime Marinated Lentils 182

    Savory Chickpea Pancake with Spinach and Sun-Dried Tomato. 184

    Wild Salmon with Apricots and Honey 187

    Toasted Pumpkin Seed Pesto Pasta with Balsamic Mushrooms 188

CHAPTER 5: Moonlight 191

Moonlight Energy Influencers 195

Feel Your Purpose: The Energy of Spirituality. 196

Let It Go: The Energy of Release 206

Sweet Dreams: The Energy of Sleep 216

Recipes to Nourish Your Moonlight Energy 223

    Dreamy Dandelion Tonic. 224

    Moonlight Bites 227

    Cinnamon Pear Cookies 228

    Coco-Banana Ice Cream with Salted Almond Butter Ripple 231

    Strawberry Super Seed Make-Ahead Breakfast 232

    Half Now, Half Later Smoothie. 235

Closing 237

Resources. 239

Acknowledgments 247

Introduction

FOR AS LONG AS I CAN REMEMBER, I'VE BEEN PARTICULARLY ATTUNED TO LIGHT. When I'm indoors I have a habit of flipping off switches and turning on lamps until I get the lighting in the room *just so*. And then there's the sun. I'm always settling down with my laptop or a cup of tea near sunny windows, chasing slivers of sunlight. I feel most like myself in the summer—a direct response to light that's longer, stronger, and warmer. But it wasn't until chronic illness that I learned that I had, in effect, a light emanating from my very own being. My body's own light illuminated my path out of unimaginable darkness at a moment when nothing else would. But before I could see my way, I had to learn to ignite my light.

What is your light? And what's the source of its power? You've no doubt heard the phrase "feeling lit up" uttered by a friend who was inspired, moved, or deeply connected to a thought, an object, a place, another person—you name it. When you feel flooded with light, you're experiencing inspiration, insight, beauty, or love; you're feeling exactly as and where you should be; you're emitting vitality and magnetism. Your light is your personal energy—the feeling that your presence conveys. That light brightens when you listen and respond to the inherent wisdom and power of your body, mind, emotions, and spirit. **Over time, maintaining that lit-from-within effect influences your beauty, strength, gratitude, relationships, health, and your life itself, both in day-to-day experience and all-encompassing journey.** In just one day, you encounter countless opportunities to ignite your inner light and apply its potential to transform your life experience. But so often, these opportunities

1

are missed. In the pages ahead, I'll help you create more of them as you move through each day of your life, from sunrise to moonlight. Get ready to surround yourself with more of what *lights you up*, and less of what leaves you feeling stuck, drained, lacking, and anything but authentically you. The result is a visible, palpable shift in your body, mind, emotions, and spirit that begins with energy—energy that supports beauty, healing, joy, connection, and even the health of our planet.

Read on if you're ready to ignite your light and, with it, your own journey of possibility.

FINDING YOUR ENERGY

Consider that every person, and every living thing, has its own unique energy. Some call it an aura, or qi, whereas others refer to it as your vibe, or your feel. It's all energy, and it's altogether different from the metabolic energy that powers you through your morning run. You see, your personal energy *is* you—it introduces you before you speak a single word. Your energy can strengthen positivity, success, and joy; reflect beauty and vitality; support health, and help you thrive amid the varied chapters and challenges of life. **Your energy is the power source for your inner light.** Within these pages, you'll find a blueprint for a day, and a life, filled with the inspiration and actions to better understand your own personal energy and ignite your light.

Ask a roomful of people for their definition of *energy*, and you'll receive answers that vary based on personal beliefs and life experience. Some define energy as straightforward physical endurance. Others will tell you it's the power that runs our heaters and appliances. Still others believe that energy is a divine guide. For a long time, I considered energy to be the stamina and motivation that carried me through the day, something I recharged each night as I slept. But there was another type of energy I had yet to understand. More than simply a force to accomplish my to-do list, I learned that **energy is an overlooked**

element in beauty, healing, and happiness—across races, cultures, and life experiences. Your energy is the feeling conveyed by your presence; it defines you in a way that you alone can choose.

If this interpretation of energy seems abstract or illusory, know that it's remarkably rooted in science. Human beings are quite literally bundles of energy; our bodies emit measurable electromagnetic fields (unsurprisingly, the strongest of those fields comes from the heart). The electricity of our bodies is influenced by outside electromagnetic fields given off by such devices as cell phones, televisions, and Wi-Fi routers, in addition to the magnetic field of the Earth itself. There's also eye-opening evidence that

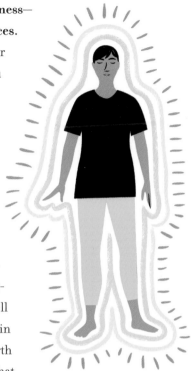

the electromagnetic fields of other people (which extend well beyond our physical bodies—estimates range from 5 to 20 feet) directly influence our own. But energy is affected by far more than just these fields. In the pages ahead, we'll explore the leading factors that impact your energy—I call them the *energy influencers*. They include mindset, movement, environment, relationships, food, spirituality—even the breaths you take. There are thirteen dynamic energy influencers to discover in this book. **Each influencer you'll encounter is like a switch that, when flipped on, floods your life with light!**

The ideas, rituals, and recipes in this book share the same key benefit of supporting the energetic health of your body. They do so in varied ways—some by shifting the actual electricity that flows throughout your body, others by rewiring habitual thought patterns, others by nourishing your body with high-quality fuel, and still others by reducing stressors that impair your body's ability to thrive at its energetic best. These energy sources work together to transform the way you look, feel, respond, and experience life. You'll find that, incorporated into your lifestyle where they feel inspiring and well suited to you, even small shifts yield major changes over days, weeks, and months. And as you change your energy over time, your whole body is also being remade, right down to the cellular level, allowing those changes to build on one another. In these pages, you'll discover that the very same energy of the body, mind, emotions, and spirit that supports healing also builds radiance. The same energy that builds radiance also grows joy. And the same energy that grows joy ignites a light in all of us, universally. Not only do you feel it personally, but others take note of it as well. Energetic shifts alter relationships, communication, and connection.

Taking care of your body with particular habits and foods might feel like a basic self-care practice that you've explored already. But look again—the ideas in this book do more for your personal energy than getting a pedicure or buying yourself a new outfit, since the effects are cumulative, and they happen on a deeper level. Your energy has the power to strengthen health, change the way your genes perform, slow the aging process, grow your happiness, and make positivity a default rather than an anomaly. **As you begin to regularly incorporate the ideas in this book, the results you'll experience may appear as a new outlook, a fresh burst of creativity, a surge of health and radiance, a feeling of renewal after a difficult time, or even the drive to change the energy of your world.** And the potential doesn't stop there—changing your energy can even alter the course of your life, enabling you to pursue big dreams and find your path to fulfill a higher purpose.

How do you know that you're ready for a personal energy shift?

You're feeling low.

You've lost your glow or your vitality.

You need to heal—physically, emotionally.

You seek more inspiration and beauty in your daily life.

You're in a rut.

You're feeling confused or adrift.

You're looking for a more meaningful approach to self-care and fulfillment.

You're feeling helpless to change negativity and pain in the world around you.

So, why hasn't this approach to energy been outlined for you before? How can something as profound as energy go unseen and unacknowledged in the majority of our daily lives? Why, at a moment when juice shops and fitness studios mark every corner, when the pursuit of wellness is undeniably mainstream, does this incredibly vital and profound aspect of our health—our energy—still feel so hazy and misunderstood?

Awareness of the body's energy has been developing for thousands of years, often on the periphery of medicine and healing. It's not typically the first place we in the Western world look to assess ourselves (preferring to take more visible or quantifiable measurements of our well-being, such as weight, physical appearance, blood pressure, or BMI). Energy is invisible and not readily measured without sophisticated tools, so it's not a familiar marker to most of us. **But everyone—and everything—around us has energy and exists in constant vibration and oscillation, even if it appears static to the eye.** As energetic healing therapies, like acupuncture, reflexology, and Reiki, continue to gain authority and visibility, we've begun to more widely acknowledge the energy that exists around us and within us, right here and right now, casting powerful

5

influence over every aspect of our lives. For many of us, not fully understanding or being able to quantify energy makes it easier to dismiss. But so many already do acknowledge the significance of energy—especially when they notice it at work in their own lives. Energy awareness often brings with it a profound shift in perspective, like a veil that lifts to reveal a previously unseen dimension of being. In the process, this awareness forges an important connection to and awareness of your body, mind, emotions, and spirit.

MY LESSONS IN THE DARK

For me, energy became a force for change, growth, healing, beauty, and joy when chronic illness threatened my life and everything I took for granted about my body—things like my ability to walk down the street, to go to the grocery store, pick up my toddler, get out of bed in the morning, or even speak without intensely discomforting, debilitating symptoms. In the process of attacking my brain and body, long-undiagnosed Lyme disease and mold exposure severely damaged my nervous and limbic systems, turning everyday experiences, such as shopping, driving, or interacting in public, into traumatic events. If you've ever had a panic attack, you know the feeling of a racing, fluttering heart (with no warning, mine likes to pop into bouts of 240 beats per minute and stay there for an hour or more), crushing anxiety, and the inability to take a full breath; this was paired with nausea and piercing stomach pain, profound weakness and fatigue; tensing, aching muscles; vision, memory, and cognition issues; sweats and extreme coldness—this state had, overnight, become my daily normal in wake, and often in sleep.

For years, there was no explanation, and then came a diagnosis—late-stage Lyme disease and coinfections—yet no clear path to healing. Those unfathomably challenging and truly surreal years deconstructed my life as I knew it, rendering every passing week darker and more desperate. For years it felt as if I lived at the bottom of an abyss without a single foothold to begin the long climb out. Still, my long search for healing became the gift, one disguised as an incredibly dark experience, that reminded me of the one function I could never lose: my ability to create my own story, led by the energy of my body.

Looking back, it's clear to me that I wouldn't have taken full ownership of my light without the dark. Before chronic illness, I was fully focused on my work as a nutrition-based beauty expert and health coach, empowering women to use food and self-care practices to look and feel their best. My *Eat Pretty* books were sharing my message with women around the globe, and I was living my own advice, having cleared my own skin and changed my body with a mix of nourishing foods and rituals. As a health coach, the healing essentials of high-quality nutrition, stress reduction, and restorative sleep had been pillars of my life for years. But chronic illness challenged everything I knew and believed about wellness, showing me that a resilient body, a joyful existence, and a strong light required even more in times of adversity. I had no choice but to look beyond my physical body to jump-start my own capacity to heal. Connecting to my energy restored a precious measure of agency over my experience and my own story that I had lost when other healing methods fell short.

In the process I discovered profound therapeutic power in major energy influencers, including connection, spirituality, mindset, and play, which I had relied on only superficially before I needed to fight for my life. In fact, the turning points in my healing journey centered on energy—especially the mindset I maintained in the difficult years before my diagnosis and during the slow, years-long fight toward remission. In a seemingly powerless place, I held onto the one power I would always possess—my energy—and with it, I reclaimed my chance to write my story on my terms. For me, the difference between being lost in painful circumstances and being moved to find the beauty around them was energy. The difference between celebrating a single step of progress rather than focusing on the miles that lay ahead was energy. In a physical body that left me feeling trapped, energy was one aspect of my life that I could fully own. And when, with my energy in mind, I resolved to seek more beauty, more of what lifted me up and made me feel resilient, and more of what enabled me to feel joy again, I took an incredibly important step to reclaim my life and my health.

Flipping my perspective to see that that the events of our lives often happen *for* us, rather than to us, further helped me to own my energetic power. Our life experiences always present opportunities for growth and change, and the toughest decisions and most challenging times can create the biggest transformation. We decide how to respond to and learn from them in turn. In this way our energy writes our stories even more directly than our circumstances. I'll admit, it's simultaneously terrifying and exciting, overwhelming and freeing, to adopt this perspective. But it's absolutely life-changing, physically, mentally, emotionally, and spiritually. It's in this space that drenching rain becomes a precious resource to enable flowers to bloom, that a forest fire creates a nutrient-dense blank canvas for rebirth, and that the darkest night makes the following morning's sunrise look like the very brightest you've ever seen.

My goal in these pages is not to motivate you to find a rainbow behind every dark cloud. I don't see myself as a self-help author who promises to share the formula for lifelong ease and success. But I do want you to become more aware of the role of energy in your life, and to experience the incredible changes that happen when you take ownership of it. I want you to feel the power you have—a power that doesn't require money, status, or any other prerequisite—to feel joyful, resilient, and lit from within throughout your life, as is your birthright. At moments this will feel easy, and at other times it will require major perseverance. **One thing is certain: your power to change your energy may actually be its most valuable at the very moment it takes the greatest courage to use.** Challenges are the chrysalis of life—transformational moments that present both the biggest unknown and the biggest potential reward in return. And the darkest times, in our lives and on our planet, can split that chrysalis wide open to reveal major beauty inside.

THE ROLES OF ENERGY IN YOUR LIFE

All along my journey, I felt that there needed to be a bigger, more open conversation about energy, in part because it answers big questions that run through so many of our minds daily. What creates beauty, attraction and magnetism, beyond our physical traits? What exactly is it that enables a body to heal? What is one tool we all possess that can make a profoundly positive shift in the world, creating a better place for us all? The answer to all of these questions involves *energy*. The energy of you, the energy of me. I want you to view your energy as a transformative tool—yet untapped, perhaps—to help you glow, heal, thrive, and boost the joy and contentment in your life. Here are just a few of the many roles that energy may play in your life:

Energy Is Beauty

As a beauty editor and health coach, I've spent my career trying to pinpoint exactly what creates our radiance and magnetism. Every one of us knows someone who seems to glow from within, whose presence we love to be in, and who leaves us feeling lighter and calmer in an "I'll-have-what-she's-having" kind of way. What is it that conveys such an extraordinary breed of beauty? It's not a symmetrical face or an hourglass body shape—just two of the many assessments of "beauty" that fall far short of capturing its essence. I'd argue that the quality we call beauty has its foundation in our personal energy. And what's more, the you that comes across in person can be vastly different from the you that comes through in a photograph, because of your energy. We're drawn to energetic qualities like joy, vibrancy, and vitality that make us feel lit from within as much as we are to strictly physical traits. When it comes to making long-term choices about life partners or friends, energy—in the form of chemistry—becomes an invisible guide.

If you find it hard to wrap your head around the overlap between energy and beauty, think of it this way: Can your energy make you happier? Absolutely.

Can your energy make you healthier? One hundred percent. And if your energy makes you both happier and healthier, there's no question that it reflects in the beauty of both your physical appearance and presence. In the pages ahead, we'll connect your energetic health to the beauty that others see in you. And we'll look even further because **at this moment there's a clear opportunity—many would say a great need—to shift our focus from physical beauty to energetic beauty—for ourselves, and for our planet.** You may feel it too: an urge to move away from a solely physical definition of yourself to something that is deeper, or more fully encompassing of the beauty of your whole being.

Energy Is Healing

If you're on a healing journey, so much of the process is in your own hands. And because wellness isn't one size fits all, our individual paths to health look different for each one of us. Many of us don't know where to start when it comes to at-home healing practices beyond food, water, exercise, and rest—and that's exactly where this book picks up, to show you that **the deepest healing often happens at the energetic level.**

Even though we all heal and thrive using different tools, there are universal ways to use energy to support these processes. This book is brimming with healing therapies, each intended to serve as a comforting, supportive embrace for a body that was designed, from the very first moment of its creation, to thrive. Beyond physical healing, shifting energy can help us restore emotionally, making it easier to forgive and prevent your beautiful spirit from being weighed down with negative experiences along the way. I hope you'll be eager to try all of the healing ideas that follow, discover what works for you, and supercharge your own health and healing capacity.

Energy Is Joy

Thoughts and moods (which, when repeated, have the power to reprogram the pathways of your brain, thanks to neuroplasticity) can be altered with small shifts. A flower in a vase by your bedside, a home-cooked meal, a supportive touch, time spent with a loved one, or consciously soaking in a happy experience are all tiny pathways to change your brain and your energy by repeatedly prompting joyous feelings—and they'll light you up in the process. Scientific study has shown us that joy gives us a healthier physical body (directly demonstrated in a healthier heart), a boost in beauty (as the stress-driven aging process slows and more resources are directed toward the skin), and even a longer life in which to share our light. Of course, feeling joy doesn't require a perfect life. Finding genuine satisfaction and sustained joy in the messy, imperfect experience of life happens when you care for your personal energy. Those who make the connection between their moods, mindset, and the energy in their lives know that there are always ways to let light in.

Energy Is Inspiration

Becoming more aware of your personal energy can reveal the parts of your life that most effectively light you up, and in the process illuminate your best course and inspire confident action. Are you seeking motivation to pursue a new project, or looking for the steps you need to take to get there? Maybe you're still searching for the opportunity or the path that you believe fits you best. If you're feeling lost or aimless, consider this book an energetic guide to the various tools that can help you find your way. The bonus: as you shift your energy you may also feel more aware of your needs and in touch with your authentic self, so that future decisions and directions flow more naturally. There's real evidence that the energetic shifts that ignite your light create mental and emotional changes, as your heart sends signals to your brain that improve the function of brain centers related to creativity, performance, and decision making.

Energy Is Nourishment

Building optimal energy means nourishing your body, mind, emotions, and spirit—with food, as well as without it. Our energy is strongly influenced by food, which literally remakes our body, molecule by molecule, after we eat. The nourishment you get from food also extends beyond nutrients to the energy of your relationship with food, the energy that your food takes on as it's prepared, and the context in which it's eaten. You'll find pages of colorful recipes woven throughout the chapters ahead, created with the goal of brightening your energy as you choose ingredients, prepare, and eat them. You'll also broaden your views on what nourishment can be, including fulfilling relationships, work, connection to the Earth, spirituality, sunlight, and a body that moves, breathes, and rests well to maintain its energetic health. Ahead, we'll explore energy on and off of your plate to find what truly satisfies you and lights you up.

Energy Is Connection

There's way more to a body than what meets the eye. When you look at a person, you can't see her emotions, you can't feel the rhythm of her heart, or see the air entering and exiting her lungs. You can't feel what it's like to be inside her body—nor can you see the energetic field that surrounds her. But you can often *sense* it. One of the best measures of your energy comes from the way others respond to your presence. What do others find in you, even before you've spoken a word? Ask your most honest friends, and you'll be amazed at the depth of what you discover. And that's only the beginning of person-to-person energetic connections. The energetic principle of "like attracts like" tells us that our energy can help us attract people and situations that bring similar energy into our lives. It's a welcome energetic collective that extends into the world around us, since we're all (yes, *all*) energetically connected. (Read more in Chapter 1.) Reason enough to bring a friend along on this journey.

Energy Is Contagious

You are an energy conduit. Whether you're aware of it or not, your energy affects everyone around you. As you practice growing your own light, it becomes easier to actively release love, joy, strength, and compassion, and watch it freely flow to others. You may be filled with the desire, and the ability, to practice random acts of kindness. To love abundantly. To care deeply for others and develop your empathetic qualities. And to lift others up to help them spark their own energetic shift. It doesn't matter how you give, to whom, or on what scale. Spreading your light is a catalyst for change in others, as well as yourself. A compliment or kind word that you say to someone else becomes both part of you and part of the person who receives it. Those words create an energetic shift in both of you, powering two lights instead of one. You'll begin to notice that whenever you spread bright energy, there's more of it to be found.

WHAT LIES AHEAD

Although the energy of our bodies is a developing frontier of research, so much of this subject has yet to be explained in scientific terms. While it feels frustrating that we don't yet have a universal way to measure, or fully comprehend, the energy of our bodies, we can still connect with its potential. Shifting your energy requires only curiosity, openness (perhaps trying activities or approaches that you've never considered), and self-reflection to discover what works for you. Know that this journey will illuminate so much more about yourself. What could an energetic shift change in your life?

During my research and writing, I spent a lot (I mean a *lot*) of time debunking unsubstantiated claims about energy. You know, the stuff you see while scrolling through your social media feeds. In this book, I favor information that can be demonstrated or proven in scientific study. However, when it comes to energy it's also true that not everything is tangible, measurable, or clear-cut. Sometimes we can base our understanding in scientific explanation (e.g., every object has a vibration; items in close proximity often begin to vibrate together), but occasionally in these pages you'll find insights that have been gleaned from anecdotal evidence, tradition, and personal experience or observations. There's clearly still so much about energy that we don't understand, that science cannot yet explain and possibly never will. And that leaves so much exciting space for exploration.

In these pages, I've chosen to include what I find to be the strongest and best-researched information on energy and methods for shifting it in your favor. And I will continue to eagerly follow developments in energy healing and energy science and share them with you on social media and in my coaching work as I apply them to my own life. In the meantime, we can approach the many gray areas of energy as "what ifs." What if water had memory? What if we could photograph energy-revealing images of plants, people, and objects? Perhaps someday these abilities will be proven or invented. Until then, don't let the number of yet-to-be-substantiated beliefs about energy sour you on its many concrete and compelling aspects.

The path to igniting your light is one that I assembled from many different influences. I think it reflects a modern approach to spirituality, beauty, wellness, and a life well lived. I hope you come to feel the same way as you read. How you use your energy will be up to you. This book is by no means the only resource you'll find on energy. We all have a slightly different experience of the phenomenon; I believe that nobody knows it all, and that you know your body best. Your personal experience with energy may be different than mine. But **whether you view energy through the lens of the spiritual, the magical, or the scientific, my goal is for you to appreciate its role as a guiding force in your life, along with your power to change it.** You will likely transcend these pages, adding exercises, affirmations, and support you find in other places. But don't be persuaded that you need special training, expensive tools, or access to healers to take hold of the power of your own energy. It's free, and yours to claim.

Ignite Your Light is about building a beautiful life, and finding your best sources of joy, healing, and energy in the process, from sunrise to moonlight. It might be a new light dawning for you—a lightbulb that turns on full of fresh ideas and inspiration. It might be a light at the end of a tunnel, helping you see yourself out of a period of darkness. Or it may serve as a spark or lightning bolt that sets some of your old ways ablaze so as to make space for new life to sprout and grow. In all of these ways and more, I hope this book will help you light yourself up from within to bring more beauty into your life and allow you to be a source of welcome energy in the world. Your end goal is not to create a life that looks good on the surface, or strive for unattainable perfection. Your goal is to ignite the light within you that makes your journey and your process the most joyful, and meaningful it can be. I hope you'll start it all anew with tomorrow's sunrise.

In beauty and health,
—Jolene

PART ONE

The Energy of You and Me

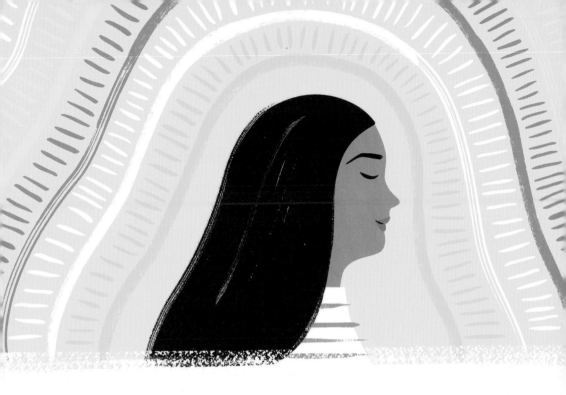

chapter one

Be the Light You Want to See

Energy informs you—and your world.

What if I told you that we share a superpower, one that's free and available to access at any moment of our lives? Your superpower, and mine, is the ability to shift the energy of your body, mind, spirit, and emotions—and in doing so consciously direct the way you experience life. You are constantly, in every moment, choosing your energy. Sure, you're being influenced by countless other energy sources (you'll get to know a ton in this book), but you're the boss of your own, giving you the ultimate authority. Even in a situation that you're helpless to change, you choose how to respond, and how you treat yourself and others in light of it. When it comes to your energy, those choices are everything. **Over time, the moment-to-moment energetic decisions you make give form to your life, connecting you to people, places, feelings, and opportunities. In the process, you also define your light.** Wherever you are in your life today, you have the ability to be a light for yourself and for the world around you. Yes, you already have the light you've been seeking. As you begin to take ownership of your energy, you'll use it to illuminate your most beautiful, resilient, and joyful self.

In this chapter, you'll find a blueprint for energetic change, which you can put into to practice today and each day forward. Start here to learn more about your energy, then take the quiz at the end of this chapter to pinpoint the part of your day to explore first for the biggest energetic power surge. Or simply follow the linear path of this book and begin with Sunrise. Progress at your own pace. There's no push to become a bright, shining beacon of endless positivity overnight (or ever, for that matter), so take time to question how this perspective works in your life and how it changes your story—past, present, and future. Once you begin to recognize how real and influential the invisible force of energy is in the world, I believe that so much of this information will come alive for you. To begin, let's look a little closer at the nature of energy, and why science already shows that it can do far more than just change the way you feel. Keep an open mind, and I know this will rock your world.

YOUR ENERGY IS:

✳ A fresh approach to recharging and refueling your body

✳ Your most important reason to prioritize self-care

✳ A new way to think about giving back

✳ A deeper understanding of beauty and the way you age

✳ An overlooked catalyst for healing

✳ A connection between you and the world'

✳ Your truest self

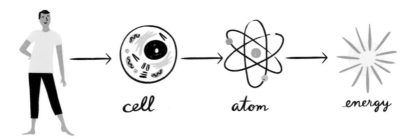

cell   atom   energy

The Physics of Energy

The science of physics explains how everything, ourselves included, is made of energy at its base level. Physicist Albert Einstein famously found in his Theory of Relativity that $E = mc^2$, which essentially shows that energy and matter are two expressions of the same substance—the stuff of which we are all composed. We may be physical beings made of cells, but those cells are comprised of atoms, which are themselves comprised of—wait for it—energy. The closer you look at an atom, the more you see that there is nothing truly material or physical within it. The solid material world that we think of as true and fundamental is, in many ways, an illusion. Wild, right? I know that it's a bit baffling to fully conceive of the energetic nature of the chair that's currently holding you up, or the glass you're drinking from, or your body as a whole. But know that the energy-filled atoms that make up matter repel each other like superstrong magnets, and that's what creates the suspension you feel as you sit on that piece of furniture or sip from that glass.

So, what exactly does this mean to be made of energy, and how does it impact our day-to-day health and happiness? Well, in many ways we're still figuring out how to apply this pretty surreal information about energy to our very real lives. Some interpret the understanding that we're all made of energy to mean that we also have the potential to shape our own reality by consciously altering our energetic building blocks—which is not nearly as complicated as it sounds. See, **we alter our energetic building blocks with every thought, action, belief, or interaction that affects our energy.** And because our bodies are constantly being remade, today's choices are the foundation of that process, and the foundation of how we experience life from this moment forward. Scientifically speaking, your energy starts to change the very moment you become conscious of it, a phenomenon called the "observer effect." The observer effect shows us that the simple act of observing allows us to have an effect on the outcome of what is being observed, as we become a part of what's happening. This means that even if you're just conceiving of your personal energy for the very first time today, you've already begun to take ownership of your superpower.

The ability to consciously direct your energy can change your life, as it exists right now, in countless ways. Energy is not static; we transform it, replenish it, and in doing so alter our body's function, activate our immune system, spark a mental or emotional shift, and change our vibration, all by choice. I can't overstate how powerful your own energetic choices are—yet so many of us fail to recognize, or act on, this potential. **The energy you choose for your body, mind,**

emotions, and spirit has a sweeping effect on every part of your life, from your physical body and beauty to the level of joy and connectedness you feel in your day-to-day existence.

Scientific study has documented that emotions and feelings have the power to alter the electromagnetic frequencies of our cells, the effects of which are felt body-wide. Take this example: The energy of your emotions affects the cardiac rhythm of your heart, which in turn causes a change in the electromagnetic frequency of your cells and directly communicates with your brain. The new electromagnetic waves emitted have an effect on your entire being, changing your energy and contributing to your heart's major role as a so-called synchronizing signal in your body.

Energy Words

The energy that makes up our bodies and everything around us is constantly in vibrating movement, giving us all that "vibe" that you've likely heard of in reference to your personal energy. And as you may have experienced, the energetic vibration of people, places, and objects you encounter has an effect on your own energy field. I find it fascinating that being in close contact with another person can bring your vibrations together, as some objects that spend time in close proximity have the tendency to vibrate together, or resonate! One breathtaking example of resonance occurs when certain species of fireflies start flashing their lights in sync as they gather in large numbers.

When we talk about energy, the vibrations of specific emotions, objects, states of health, and the like are often labeled "high vibe" or "'low vibe." This refers to the assumption that "high vibe" energy is lighter and freer, whereas "low vibe" energy is heavy and burdensome. Truthfully, I find these labels to be a bit misleading and even confusing because we still simply don't *know* their vibrations. There's not a specific vibration or vibrational range we can truly aspire to, because we just don't understand vibrations in such a straightforward way yet. Some experts have already begun to measure vibration and I have no doubt that this will continue to be a fascinating area of scientific exploration in decades to come. But right now, here in this book, I won't be using "high vibe" or "low vibe" to describe energy.

In their place, I use words that describe light—"bright energy" and "dim energy"—to discuss the overall spectrum of effects that the energy influencers in our lives have on the way we feel, the way we look, and the way we respond to and experience life. You can be the judge of what brightens or dims your light, simply by feeling. So, when certain people, places, objects, or emotions hit you smack in the head or heart with a big "Yes!" seek more of those things.

Rather than position energy states as polarities, like good or bad, positive or negative, I view the varied energy states we experience as parts of the same whole. All energy is information. Passing between energetic states is like tuning the dial on a car radio, or adjusting lighting with a dimmer switch, rather than completely switching on or off. Calling some energy "positive" and other energy "negative" sounds a lot like I'm telling you that what you're experiencing is good or bad, rather than you just learning to use energy as your guide. So, in this book, I also avoid using "positive" and "negative" as much as possible and instead reference what is likely to brighten or dim your light. Feeling the whole spectrum of energy is a part of life—it creates a yin/yang balance. **States of dim energy enable us to fully experience bright energy. And as you tune between them, you're already shifting your inner light, and owning your superpower.**

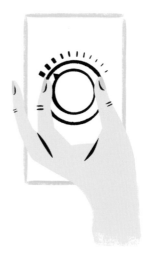

DIM ENERGY

What does it actually feel like to experience bright or dim energy? Although you've shifted between these energetic states thousands of times before, these descriptive words might help you see and feel your energy in a new light.

Dim energetic states may leave you feeling:

Anxious	*Apathetic*	*Cheated*
Fearful	*Judgmental*	*Short-tempered*
Sad	*Uninspired*	*Selfish*
Jealous	*Angry*	*Lackluster*
Confused	*Worried*	*Dejected*
Stressed	*Unfocused*	*Stuck*
Unwell	*Disconnected*	*Pessimistic*
Self-pitying	*Unhappy*	*Unsettled*

You can probably imagine what it's like to be led by dim energy. Imagine you're reading a book outside as the sun goes down and it gradually gets darker. Without a light source, it's not as easy to decipher the sentences. Words get mixed up. In your life, dim energy often translates to a murkier perspective than you'd have with bright energy illuminating your path and connecting you to your essence, inspiring you to use your power and potential, and helping you move toward your deepest desires. In dim energetic states, like jealousy, self-pity, and fear, your perspective is clouded, and so often what you see is only those immediate feelings. Dim energy truly dulls your ability to see and even to receive hope, beauty, possibility, and love. Over time, existing in a state of dim energy and its clouded worldview bring on the very real deleterious physical effects of sustained negative emotions. Stress and negativity beget prolonged high cortisol in the body, which breaks down collagen in your skin, contributes to unwanted weight gain (high cortisol is specifically connected to extra abdominal weight), makes it harder to get restorative sleep, speeds up the aging process, and suppresses your immune system, among other effects. Anger in particular is linked to anxiety, insomnia, fatigue, brain fog, low self-esteem, and even increased risk of infection or illness, as your immune system is weakened for about six hours after simply recalling an angry experience.

Overall, dim energy depletes your physical health and beauty in addition to hanging a cloud over your mindset and emotions. And the more time you spend in those dim energetic places, natural as they may be, the more you train your brain and body to live in that space, suppressing your immune system—and happiness—in the process. Although dim energy isn't something you can or need to wholly avoid, you may want to make an effort to shift or replace some of the dim energy sources in your daily life because of the limits they place on your body, mind, emotions, or spirit. Think: thoughts, people, places, or even media. It's more than okay to do this, especially while you're actively working to change your energy. Most sadness, fear, anxiety, and the like are normal human emotions, so spot them when they arrive, let yourself feel them, and then release them with the knowledge that those energy states can actually be a form of guidance or intuition.

So many of the dim energy inputs we encounter each day aren't valuable or necessary, so aim to pinpoint those and limit them. Consider the upsetting show you binge-watched last night or the co-worker who wants you to join her to gossip about the rest of your office. Sometimes removing dim energy from your life is the simplest way to see and feel a difference without changing anything else at all. Although I'm definitely not advocating that you force or fake the appearance of happiness, confidence, optimism, or any other bright energy state, if you can identify what is diminishing your light, it serves you to remove yourself from it. And when you separate from that which is obscuring your brilliance, how brightly will you shine? How amazing will you feel? How renewed will your routine become? Only you can decide to find out.

Committing to brighter energy more of the time allowed me to support physical and emotional healing and climb toward wholeness, one energetic shift at a time. But healing or change is not always linear. Even as I worked to brighten my energy, I very regularly had days where I wanted to scream, cry, and just be with the emotional pain of my experience. I gave, and continue to give, myself full permission to feel those emotions, doing my best to release them in a way that supports my health, and then looking forward to waking up the next day feeling one small step brighter. I hope you'll see that possibility in your own journey, whether you want to change yourself or change your world.

NEGATIVITY BIAS

If it seems far easier to see the proverbial glass of life as half empty, you may just be feeling a natural biological instinct called the negativity bias. This is the tendency of your brain and body to react more intensely to negative stimuli and more readily store negative memories—a protective mechanism that evolved to keep us from harm. It's estimated that our bodies place three times more significance on negative events and emotions than on positive ones. Simply put, this means that when something sad, embarrassing, painful, or upsetting happens, we don't forget it easily. We may have to work a little harder to steer our energy toward what's bright, but I think the potential to change your brain, body, and biology in the process is more than worth the effort.

BRIGHT ENERGY

When you're emitting bright energy, it often feels as if all of your senses become heightened. You see clearly and notice more beauty; you hear even the whispers of your heart; you connect to others more easily; and you feel the energy of people, places, and objects that perhaps went unnoticed before. When you have ample bright energy flooding you from different areas of your life, you feel *lit from within*. As your light continues to brighten, so much is illuminated.

Just like dim energy, bright energy has physical effects—think a surge of immune system activity, release of feel-good neurotransmitters, and more stable hormone levels over time. Simply feeling joy releases dopamine and serotonin that further enhance health and happiness. And feeling content and relaxed reduces muscle tension (allowing for increased circulation and glow to your skin), supports skin healing, helps maintain balanced blood sugar and hormones that support so many aspects of health, and improves digestion and nutrient absorption, which fuels your body from the inside out. That's not to mention the positive changes to your mood, memory, and ability to focus.

Bright energetic states may leave you feeling:

Joyful	*Empathetic*	*Optimistic*
Hopeful	*Content*	*Peaceful*
Motivated	*Beautiful*	*Strong*
Loving	*Healthy*	*Clear*
Inspired	*In the flow*	*Grateful*
Generous	*Balanced*	*Patient*
Resilient	*Fulfilled*	*Creative*
Compassionate	*Connected*	*Grounded*

At some point, you may wonder—could your energy be *too* bright? If you're forcing yourself to feel bright energy all of the time, you may be ignoring other energy and emotions that could help protect or guide you. By limiting your focus to light alone, you're only taking in one side of the whole. The way I experience it, you can stay lit up enough to strongly support your beauty, resilience, and joy without needing to project bright energy 24/7. We all have days, weeks, years even, when our energy gets dimmed, and it's more than okay to experience those times with the knowledge that you can once again tune back to brightness.

In reality, we all vacillate between bright and dim energy over the course of an average day. I want to help you spend more of your time solidly in the bright energy space, and to see how the shift from dim to bright changes your day-to-day life. The results will be visible: in your skin and the health of your body; palpable: in your mood and your motivation; and transformative: in your life, your relationships, and your overall joy.

VIBRATION AND ITS LINK TO CONSCIOUSNESS

If all matter vibrates, why do we, as humans, possess a more sophisticated ability to think, feel, and have self-awareness than, say, a grain (or mountain) of sand? One of the latest theories about vibration and consciousness posits that human beings achieve large-scale "macro-consciousness" through the combined energy of the huge number of "micro-conscious" parts of our body, each of which has its own vibration. All of those individual, simple vibrations (the ones that look similar to that possessed by a grain of sand) create a being that's extremely complex when those independent vibrations begin to work together, or resonate. This is known as the resonance theory of consciousness, and it's one of many fascinating theories about how human consciousness works.

UNIVERSAL CONNECTION

Quantum mechanics shows us how everything and everybody may be connected, in a theory called quantum entanglement. Quantum entanglement demonstrates that the tiny particles that make up energy become connected, or entangled, with each other when they come into contact, and then subsequently remain entangled even when separated across great distances. Applying this to our lives, it means that the separation that we feel from one another may only be a perception, not reality. Einstein called this feeling of separation an "optical delusion." This theory illustrates one reason energy is so powerful in creating our reality and in building an energetic movement much larger than ourselves. Researchers have also hypothesized that human energy and consciousness affect us all globally via the Earth's magnetic field, which creates a feedback loop with the magnetic fields surrounding human brains and hearts. By consciously choosing your own energy, you may in fact be promoting a universal shift.

Where Is Your Energy?

When we discuss the light energy of the body in this book, we'll refer to four distinct areas of focus: body, mind, emotions, and spirit. Sorting your energy into these four facets not only grows your awareness of the role each area plays in your energetic life, it helps you understand why something that appears to affect just one facet of your energy can in fact influence all four.

ENERGY OF YOUR BODY

When it comes to your body, supporting and renewing energy has its foundation in the essential health practices that you've been taught since childhood: good nutrition, ample water, physical activity, proper hygiene (think: brushing and flossing), adequate rest. When you don't check these boxes regularly, you run the risk of depleting the physical components of your one precious body. As an adult, you take the basic tenets of physical wellness that you learn in childhood and learn to apply them to your unique self. For you, "good nutrition" might become a low-sugar diet that decreases inflammation, or it might be a daily superfood smoothie that feeds your body.

Physical activity might come from the stand-up treadmill desk you install in your office, or the afternoon break you take for circuit training. Not all health practices affect each of us in the same way, so pay attention to your own personal essentials to create your optimal body energy. You'll learn in this book that you can care for and improve the health of your body by consciously brightening the energy of your mind, emotions, and spirit as well, since all four are parts of one whole. Many issues that appear to be limited to the physical body have their roots in one of your other three energy facets.

Your body energy needs more support if you experience:

* **Regular fatigue**

* **That "hangry" feeling, often caused by blood sugar imbalances**

* **Frequent illness**

* **Aches and pains with no clear cause**

* **Unresolved skin issues**

* **Digestive upset**

For your body energy, pay special attention to Energy of Movement (page 70), Energy of Food (page 49), and Energy of Sleep (page 216).

ENERGY OF YOUR MIND

If you made an honest list of everything that's currently on your mind—tonight's dinner, the conference call you have in fifteen minutes, next week's trip, the haircut you need to schedule, your friend's birthday, the workout you want to fit in later today, and the list goes on—I bet you'd be shocked at just how much your mind juggles at any given moment. Just because you *can* juggle an extensive number of items at once doesn't mean that it's beneficial to do so. **A mind that's constantly overwhelmed is one of the most overlooked energy drains in our modern world; it damages your physical health, emotions, and spirit just as much as your mental function.** Practices that encourage extended mental focus, as well as freedom or space for ideas, invention, and feeling present, can breathe new energy into your mind, while lowering your stress, improving mental performance, and supporting digestion and blood sugar balance. We'll look at many of those ahead.

Your mind energy needs more support if you experience:

* **Inability to concentrate**
* **Slow thinking and response time**
* **Insomnia due to a racing mind**
* **Memory problems**
* **Creative blocks**
* **Brain fog**

For your mind energy, pay special attention to Energy of Work and Creativity (page 105).

ENERGY OF YOUR EMOTIONS

Emotional ups and downs are part of life's learning experience. No one can be calm, positive, and composed *all the time*. But your default emotional state, the place your emotions go when you have time out to reset, is important to look at as a barometer of your emotional energy. If your default emotions follow an energy-depleting pattern, such as cycling through worry, anger, or lack, this reflects the energy you give attention to on a regular basis. And those dim emotional states, as you might have guessed, have been shown to compromise your ability to perform and focus, to act in a leadership capacity, to maintain good health, even to see your own value in the world and rise to your highest purpose.

Change your emotional patterns, including the way you manage and respond to your emotions, however, and you can expand your ability to focus and create, as well as lower physical markers of poor health, such as inflammation. Emotions, though they are felt, are also believed to be stored within your physical body during highly emotional experiences in your life—that is, until you actively release them. You may be able to pinpoint a place where you feel an emotion in your body right now. As you recognize and acknowledge it, you begin to express and help release it. Your emotions are signals that have tremendous impact on your energy and your inner light, especially relative to the way that light affects others. Practices like gratitude, time out to reset your emotions, and drawing out the feeling of positive emotions can elevate your emotional state and build the energy you want; we'll explore more of these ahead.

Your emotional energy needs more support if you experience:

* **Defaulting to one emotional extreme, like frequent crying or anger**

* **Inability to handle stress**

* **Being easily triggered to explosive emotions**

* **Allowing others to control your emotions**

For your emotional energy, pay special attention to Energy of Release (page 206) and Energy of Your Mindset (page 61).

ENERGY OF YOUR SPIRIT

Your energy is as connected to your spirit as it is to your physical body, although we so often judge only the physical. Your spirit energy reflects your essence, your connection to your purpose, your values, beliefs, and what (or whom) you hold dear. Spirit energy is the energetic wild card that can pull you through the toughest circumstances and guide your life in incredible ways. But it's so often ignored or untapped—until you truly need it. Connecting with the energy of your spirit, or your true self, can support you in feeling more fulfilled in your daily life, even if your routine hasn't changed. If this area of your life needs more attention, jump ahead to Chapter 5 and spend time thinking about your core beliefs, the purpose you feel in your life, and how they show up in your daily routine.

Your spirit energy needs more support if you experience:

✳ **Lack of purpose or fulfillment**   ✳ **Disconnect**

✳ **Boredom with life**   ✳ **Difficulty finding your path**

For your spirit energy, pay special attention to Energy of Spirituality (page 196).

Mapping Energy in the Body

Where is our energy? Ideally, it's everywhere within and around us, flowing and circulating freely. All the energy within and around you in your electromagnetic field is often called your energy body. The atmosphere that surrounds your body is also sometimes referred to as your aura. Within your energy body, there are established energy centers and pathways that you may hear or learn about in your exploration of energy. Here are a few to know:

CHAKRAS

The body has over a hundred energy centers called chakras, but the focus lies on the main seven that comprise an energetic spine, from the pelvic floor and base of the spine (your root chakra), up to the crown of the head (your crown chakra). As you might imagine, your root chakra is the center of energy connected to the earth, while your crown chakra connects to divine and spiritual energy. The five other chakras in between are: the sacral chakra (located in your lower abdomen), the solar plexus chakra (beneath your ribs in the center of your body), the heart chakra, the throat chakra, and the third eye chakra (between your eyebrows). Each corresponds to a color, part of the body, and aspect of your energy, and you may find them linked to certain gemstones and essential oils as well.

The chakras are especially interesting because they clearly connect health concerns or emotions with their energetic home bases in the body. I find them

34

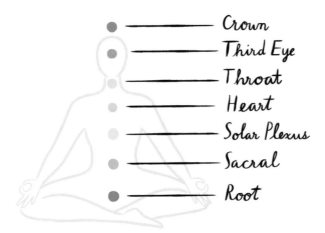

Crown
Third Eye
Throat
Heart
Solar Plexus
Sacral
Root

to be very logical, and a helpful place to begin thinking about the energy that's stored in different areas of your body. Typically, if you identify an energetic blockage in one or more of your chakras (usually pinpointed through physical symptoms or feelings unique to each chakra), you'll want to go through the process of clearing that chakra, which is a little different for each one. This is something you can do alone or guided by an energy practitioner. Just by bringing energy and consciousness to a specific chakra, you begin to support your health in that area. Because each chakra is associated with a color, finding the chakra or chakras that could use extra attention could inspire you to bring a certain color into your life through food, clothing, or other objects.

MERIDIANS

Meridians are pathways or channels through which energy flows in your body. The twelve primary meridians of the body were established centuries ago and continue to be recognized and validated for their ability to influence energy flow and health outcomes. Although meridians can't be physically located, like the components of your circulatory system, they create an energetic map of your body in much the same way.

ENERGY SENSITIVITY

What does it mean to be energetically sensitive? About 20 percent of the population appear to have slight differences in emotional and social processing, including more activity in the brain's empathy-developing mirror neurons, more difficulty tuning out stimuli due to greater alertness, and more vivid emotional experience via the prefrontal cortex—the part of the brain that processes sensory data. If you find yourself experiencing events, feelings, and energy more deeply than those around you, this could be you!

Signs that you may be particularly sensitive to energy:

※ **You need more frequent opportunities to disconnect from others.**

※ **You're sensitive to loud noises, crowded places, bright lights.**

※ **You sense the energy or moods of others, and they affect you.**

※ **You find that you need more peace and calm than others.**

※ **You experience seemingly random blood sugar lows or cravings.**

※ **You feel easily overwhelmed.**

The physiological explanation of energy sensitivity is rooted in genetics that affect the brain and nervous system and that are further influenced by your environment, especially that of your childhood. In addition, energetically sensitive people often find that their intuition seems finely tuned; another result of the brain working extra hard at emotional and social processing and creating subtle insights or feelings that others may miss.

Many energy-sensitive people find these strategies helpful:

※ **Know your limits and don't feel that you have to apologize for them.**

※ **Find places or opportunities to remove yourself when needed.**

※ **Practice energy-shifting breathing exercises.**

✳ **Meditate to clear and focus your mind.**

✳ **Be sure to eat high-quality protein and mineral-rich foods, including unrefined salts.**

✳ **Practice your own instant energy shifts (see ahead).**

Three Steps to Energetic Change

Taking charge of your personal energy is incredibly empowering. The more you grow your awareness of your energy and the more often you shift it to match the way you want to feel, the better you'll be able to guide your experience and your life in the process. A change in energy provokes a shift in who you believe you can be, the meaning you give your life, how you view and respond to your current life situation, and your deepest desires for yourself. Like a song you heard in passing that pops up again and again in your head all day, energy is an undercurrent of your life. And when you actively choose your energy, you more easily default to that pattern again and again, influencing your present and steering your future. Within you at this very moment there's immeasurable capacity to thrive, heal, and experience joy and contentment. Do you feel connected to it? Is it working in your life? If not, allow me to guide you through some of the most compelling ways to discover and activate this potential in your body, mind, emotions, and spirit. To shift your own energy in this moment, you need only to practice these three things: awareness, discovery, and expansion.

STEP 1

AWARENESS

Grow your awareness of the energy around and within you, as well as your ability to change it. Shifting energy begins with observation before action. Observing your energy is the foundational element to any change you're going to make. Start paying attention to your thoughts, actions, and reactions, without judgment.

Just the process of becoming aware starts your energetic shift (remember "the observer effect" that says observing alone changes the outcome?) and empowers you to change what's not working for you, helping you create the life you desire in the long run. Pay close attention to the energetic message that you send to those around you (and back to yourself) each day. Instead of relying on the mirror or photographs to assess your body and beauty, practice noticing your energy (don't worry, you'll only enhance your physical glow in the process).

Savor this time to recognize where and who you are today. Watch how your body responds to experiences in your day—are there changes in breathing, overwhelm, gut feelings, fears, excitement, strong likes or dislikes? This is all information. From whom, what, or where do these energetic responses arise? Make space to notice this energy in yourself, and let it show you where you can make changes. Lyme-related dysautonomia caused a state of extremely heightened nervous system for me, one that had the unexpected benefit of allowing me to be intensely in tune with energy. The more I witnessed my body's strong reactions to different energy sources, the more I could see very clearly which situations and thought patterns were placing a heavy burden on my nervous system and body while it was trying to heal. I felt drawn to focus on my inner energy to support and enhance the other external healing practices I had chosen. When I removed my personal blocks to healing energy (changing my work schedule, allowing for more rest, reducing negative stimuli, and elevating my mindset), it felt as if an immense barrier to healing had been lifted.

STEP 2

DISCOVERY

Find which people, experiences, places, thoughts, or objects brighten your energy. What truly lights you up? This should be easy to answer—yet it often isn't. In the energy discovery step of this process, identify the tools that help you maintain the energy you want every day. Grab a pencil and paper and write out a list of the bright energy sources in your life. When do you feel the most loved, or feel love toward someone or something else? Can you list ten things that help you feel joy and contentment? Twenty? Now, of that list, star the items that can be used to shift your energy instantly, at any time and in any place. Think: listening to a favorite song, reciting a mantra, doing a kind act for someone else, or sipping a favorite cup of tea. These are your instant shifts. Keep a list of them on your phone, at your desk, by your bedside, or wherever you'll see them most. And practice your instant shifts whenever you need a light in your day or a lift in your spirits.

MY INSTANT SHIFTS

Grounding my feet in the grass or sand

Listening to music I love

Changing my outfit

Taking a 15-minute nap

Meditation

Putting on makeup

Diffusing a mood-lifting essential oil

A conversation with a friend

Doing something nice for someone else

Sitting in sunlight

Snuggling or playing with my little boy

Spending time with my husband

A hot bath or a skincare ritual

Reading a book

Watching a documentary

Spending time in nature

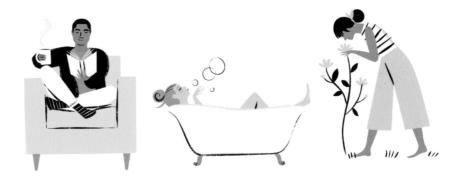

How many days go by when you don't get to do any of the things on your list? Make it your goal to not let a single day pass without having *at least one* of these experiences—try for many more. Prioritize them and pencil them in. As you do, you direct more energy toward beauty, resilience, and joy. I think you'll also notice that each bright energetic experience makes the next a little more natural. Be aware that as your energy changes, some of your items could drop off the list, and others could join.

STEP 3

EXPANSION

Expand the presence of bright energy sources in your life every day. Once you get clear on the bright energy sources in your life, incorporate them often. Practice visualizing the feeling you get from a bright energy source spreading through your body, permeating every cell, especially places where you may have physical issues or feel stuck in dim energy. Perhaps it starts in your stomach, feeling light like butterflies, and spreads gently over you with golden warmth. Extend and sink into at least one experience like this each day (try for several), and you'll use your mind to expand the energetic health of your entire being.

Next time you need to shift or replace energy, practice these three quick and extremely effective steps—I call them the three R's:

REMOVE *yourself from the person, place, thought, etc. that's dimming your energy.*

RELEASE *it from your mind. Remember that it was just a person, place, thought, etc. and it doesn't define you. You can reinforce this by practicing a form of re-lease—think: a sigh, a stretch, a prayer or mantra, journaling, etc. You'll learn many more in Chapter 5.*

RESET *your energy. Practice one of your instant shifts to brighten your energy, or simply pause where you are and call to mind an object, idea, or experience that lights you up (see my "So Good" exercise on page 76 if you need help doing this).*

40

Start small, if needed. Look around you, out the window, in the mirror, in your memory. Take a moment to feel how your chosen thought or action affects your energy, and stay with that feeling for a moment or two longer than you normally would. What makes it so good? Does that feeling have a color or emotion? Let that color or emotion sink in; remember the way it feels.

You'll never stop choosing, creating, and building your energetic reality. Your perspective is always being informed by new experiences, and perhaps changing in the process. **Remember that this ordinary-seeming moment is actually quite exceptional, as it's a chance to change your experience. Think of this very moment as the most special occasion that you have, and don't save or put off feeling beauty, resilience, and joy for tomorrow.** Your personal energy comes from all the tiny moments of building and rebalancing throughout the day, each one full of potential.

YOUR HEALTH AND THE LIMITS OF CHOICE

Let's be very clear: while you can choose your energy, you cannot choose your circumstances. And you can't, for example, choose your way out of a mental health issue, like depression or anxiety, the same way I can't choose my way out of late-stage Lyme. The thing is, you can choose your energy around it. I now view my chronic illness as a metamorphic experience that pushed me to evolve and wildly reprioritize in ways I never would have willingly chosen. The process was incredibly painful, and so much was lost—but I know now that perhaps what I once viewed as losses were not right for me in the first place. Beauty continues to come from this journey, and I know that's because I choose that outcome every day. That choice is available for you, too.

The Process

Take a look at the chapters ahead, brimming with food, habits, challenges, ideas, and rituals that spark energetic shifts. These ideas aren't all or nothing; one or two new rituals may be more deeply transformative for you than completely overhauling your daily routine.

Personally, I eased into my own energy transformation with tiny, repetitive habits. At moments when my energy felt depleted, dim, or weakened, I started making a conscious effort to incorporate the ideas in this book—and the shifts to bright energy became easier and more frequent, as if I were strengthening a muscle. Looking back, I've almost completely reshaped my daily rituals over the last few years, and I feel the difference in clarity of mind, calmness of spirit, and physical glow. It still amazes me that these changes were self-guided, and free. I am certain that I'll continue to learn more and make changes that fine-tune my energy, because our lives are never static. I hope you'll start here with me, right now, today.

So, where's the proof that the energy influencers in this book are going to make you more attractive, happier, and healthier? As in my own climb out of darkness, it will be in the connections you make, the deep breaths you take, the satisfaction with your life, and the heaviness you feel lift from your shoulders when you realize that you may not control life, but you can control your own energy in this moment. You make conscious energetic choices every day. **Your own energy is an alchemy of thoughts and feelings, food and movement, people and surroundings that are uniquely yours.** I believe that the body was made to thrive and that it possesses innate healing abilities. Our job is to support it, and to release the factors that are standing in its way—think: a stressful environment, negative beliefs and thought patterns, taxing relationships, or unfulfilling routines. I believe that we can accelerate healing, open ourselves to optimal beauty and health, and grow our joy and fulfillment by shifting the energy in our bodies and lives, thus igniting our lights. This energy comes from the natural world around us, from others, from ourselves. We have the ability to expand it in our lives and develop its power sources, changing the way we experience our day-to-day lives.

I ask that you believe in the brightness that is possible in your life when you choose it for yourself, regardless of how dark your circumstances seem or feel at times. Believe that you deserve beautiful, joyful things. Believe that you are, and have always been, resilient—even if your body, mind, emotions, and spirit have been carrying a heavy burden. You have more control—and more wisdom—than you think you do. Even in this moment you write your story, with every energetic choice.

DEFINE YOUR ENERGY QUIZ

As you develop your energy awareness, you'll likely pinpoint one or two parts of the day—Sunrise, Daylight, Sunset, or Moonlight—that could use extra focus. This Define Your Energy quiz will also guide you, by narrowing down the portion of your day that might benefit most from an energetic shift. Start with small changes, and I know you'll feel the momentum build. Look beyond the limitations of the routine you're in, and open yourself to something unfamiliar—from repainting a room to changing your career, to spending time visualizing yourself in perfect health. You'll know what you're ready for.

Check the circles that are a firm yes for you. Leave everything else blank.

SUNRISE

○ My morning thoughts set a positive tone for my day.

○ I take time to move my body as a form of waking up.

○ I set intentions for my day based on my energy, desires, and long-term goals.

○ I have daily opportunities to connect with the sun or morning light.

○ After dressing and grooming, I leave the house feeling lit up.

TOTAL CHECKED _____.

DAYLIGHT

- ○ I feel energized by what I do each day.
- ○ When I need to, I can focus on one task without interruption until it's complete.
- ○ I make time to connect in a meaningful way with colleagues, friends, or family during my day.
- ○ When I take on a project, my ideas and actions seem to flow.
- ○ Even when I'm busy, I set aside moments to check in with my body and breathing during the day.

TOTAL CHECKED _____.

SUNSET

- ○ I regularly make time for fun, playful activities.
- ○ My home environment makes me feel great when I'm there.
- ○ I bring nature inside my home with natural objects, fresh air, green plants, and ample sunlight.
- ○ I listen to or make music that fills me with bright energy.
- ○ I take time to care for myself and others in ways that bring me joy.

TOTAL CHECKED _____.

MOONLIGHT

- ○ Before bed, I let go of unwanted energy that I've accumulated during the day.
- ○ I have a spiritual practice that adds meaning to my life.
- ○ I aim to live to my highest good, for myself and for others.
- ○ I disconnect and put my devices away well before bedtime.
- ○ I fall asleep easily and rest soundly through the night.

TOTAL CHECKED _____.

What part of your day could use an energetic shift?

Compare the number of statements you checked within each of the four parts of your energetic day with the guidelines below:

Sunrise total: _____

Daylight total: _____

Sunset total: _____

Moonlight total: _____

0–1 CHECKS: Your energy is in need of a big shift during this time of day. Make this chapter a primary focus for your efforts to brighten your light and enhance beauty, resilience, and joy in your life. Get excited: your life is ripe for the transformation that comes from igniting your light with new energy!

2–3 CHECKS: Your personal energy is struggling a bit at this time of the day. Strengthening your bright energy flow with the energy influencers in this chapter will have a noticeable impact on your energy and light you up from within, making a major difference over time.

4–5 CHECKS: Your personal energy is strong at this time of the day! You're in the flow, and your life is open to experiences of beauty, resilience, and joy that continually replenish your light. Take a moment to honor yourself for the energy you've chosen in this part of your day, and resolve to bring more of this energy to other areas of your life, and the lives of others.

PART TWO

Your Energetic Day

INTRODUCTION

Welcome to the beginning of your energetic day, the place you revisit for a fresh start once every 24 hours. In the days, weeks, and months ahead, you'll use the energy influencers in the forthcoming pages to light your way to beauty, resilience, and joy. Start by accessing and appreciating the bright energy that's already in your life, then expand that energy as it works for you. Maybe you've already changed your diet, or started to meditate; perhaps you've explored energetic healing practices, or it could be that the concept of energy is all new to you. Wherever you are in your journey, there's something here to support you and light you up from within. Brightening your energy benefits so many aspects of your mind, body, and spirit—from boosting your physical glow to supporting healing to increasing your capacity to give to those around you—and I know you'll be amazed as you become more conscious of this power.

Here's what you can expect ahead:

Each of the energy influencers you'll discover in this book have been organized to fit into four parts of your day: Sunrise, Daylight, Sunset, and Moonlight. Chapter 2 will guide you through the energy of Sunrise, the earliest part of your day, from about five a.m. to nine a.m., when the energy of your mindset, movement, and the way you prepare yourself for the day makes a lasting impression on your energy. You'll connect to the sun and fresh air to experience the energy of nature in the early morning, and you'll taste some of my favorite recipes for brightening your energy at breakfast. Chapter 3 welcomes Daylight, from nine a.m. to five p.m., when the energy of work and creativity, relationships and connection, and breath are major energetic guides. You'll derive energy from the earth and plants, and find inspiration-fueling recipes for power-packed lunches and snacks during the most active part of your day. Chapter 4 transitions to Sunset, from five p.m. to nine p.m., a time to make more room for laughter, play, and music, as well as to enjoy your sacred home space—all of which strongly influence your personal energy. In this chapter, prepare to experience the energy of water and natural objects, and to find recipes that restore and nourish at a time of day when you gather with family or friends to enjoy a meal, or simply eat to replenish yourself. In Chapter 5, Moonlight arrives—the dark hours between nine p.m. and five a.m.—a moment to pause for the energy of spirituality, energetic release, and sleep. You'll connect to the energy of the moon, stars, and the dark night, and cap off your day with light, sleep-supporting sweets, snacks, and drinks.

Many of the influencers that you'll explore ahead can pop up anytime in your day, so you can view them as fluid parts of your daily experience. If you find your moments for exercise and movement in the evening rather than the morning, or you prefer to start the day with song rather than spoken words of gratitude, that's wonderful—and it's your own way. Trust your intuition and let the resulting joy and beauty that you experience be strong indicators of the personal energy shift that you've achieved. Always create the energetic day that feels best to you. And remember, you are in control of the process. You follow no one else's goals or timeline but your own.

THE ENERGY OF FOOD

Food itself is a leading influencer of your personal energy across the entire day. The acts of cooking, preparing, or simply nourishing your body weave through each of the four parts of your energetic day, and ahead you'll find food-related inspiration within each chapter. Food affects the energy of each of us a little differently, so consider which of these four main aspects of food's energy is most influential to your own:

1
THE ENERGY OF INGREDIENTS

Food is essential fuel for so many of your body's functions—fuel that breaks down to become the building blocks of your body, including your skin, hair, and nails. The food you eat literally becomes *you*, as your body completes the constant process of remaking and rebuilding itself, molecule by molecule. But not all food is created equal. You have the opportunity to influence both your physical body and your energy body with the energetic capacity of the ingredients you choose, many of which take their energy directly from the sun and earth. When you bite into ingredients grown or nourished by sunlight, for example, you're literally eating the energy of the sun's light. Sunlight creates energy in plants that we then use to make the ATP that powers our cells and bodies.

When it comes to fruit and vegetables, I find the most energetic benefit in ingredients that are just recently picked, or have only traveled short distances to get to my table. The energy of a handful of greens that I tear off straight from the garden or tomatoes that are still warm from the sun is so much greater than the same ingredients that I find in a grocery store, after they've spent days or weeks in refrigeration to reach me. I also find that I prefer the energy of some food fully cooked, and others raw or only lightly warmed—often depending on the season and the ingredient itself. And I think you'll notice that the energy of whole foods is more pronounced than that of the extracts or isolated components of foods, since whole or minimally processed foods often retain a spectrum of compounds that work together synergistically.

As you choose your food, ask some of these questions: How and where was it grown or produced? Did this ingredient have access to fresh air, sunlight, clean air and water, and rich soil or another high-quality source of energy and nutrients while it developed? What is its story; under what circumstances did it come to you, and far has it traveled?

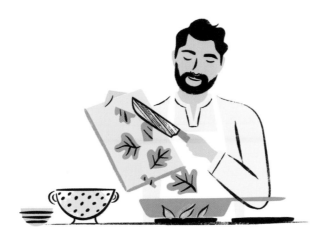

② THE ENERGY OF FOOD PREPARATION

Could the energy of Mom's home-cooked food render it more nourishing or restorative than the same store-bought version? I'm not alone in suspecting that your energy—whether bright or dim—makes its way into the food you prepare, even if you're not conscious of it. Next time you're exhausted, stressed, or annoyed at the thought of lighting up the stove, take a break and practice some instant energy shifts before getting back in the kitchen (or take the day off and hit up a restaurant you love!).

Cooking, to me, is like meditation; it allows me to enter as flow state, as well as to play—with ingredients, flavors, colors, moods. Multiple studies have shown the benefits of creativity in the kitchen, from increased confidence and happiness to alleviating anxiety and depression, or a boost in feelings of connectedness when you're cooking for others. Sure, not every meal is a joy if you're tired, stressed, or hungry. But I recognize the potential to infuse my cooking with bright, love-filled energy every time I pull out my pots, pans, and well-worn cutting boards. In the kitchen, I consciously aim to shift my energy to a brighter space, feeling gratitude for the chance to cook and eat food that supports my health and beauty.

51

❸

THE ENERGY OF YOUR FOOD
RELATIONSHIP

In my decade as a health coach, one of the most universal truths that I've found is that your personal view of food dramatically affects the way your body receives it. Brightening the energy around your relationship with food is nothing short of transformative for your body—something that I experienced firsthand when I stopped seeing food as an enemy and realized it was my most overlooked tool for beauty. And now there's even scientific evidence to support this outlook, including a study that found a difference in the way food was received by the body based on participants' beliefs about its calorie content and the health benefits of its ingredients. Incredibly, if you believe a food is healthier for you, it may actually become so. However, when food is clouded by stress, fear, or anxiety, it loses much of its healing potential. Your body is unable to even digest food properly unless it's in a relaxed, para-sympathetic state (read: free from dim energy states like worry or anger). Be aware that the energy you receive from food is influenced by your beliefs, memories, and even fears, giving it yet another level of energetic influence.

❹

THE ENERGY OF YOUR
EATING ENVIRONMENT

Think about the last meal you enjoyed. Not the last meal you *ate*—the last one you relished for amazing flavors, or special company, or a meaningful occasion. Those factors—where, why, how, and with whom your food was served and eaten—influenced the state of your energy at that meal, making your eating environment arguably as important as the food itself. The way you feel—stressed, joyful, uncomfortable, distracted—as you eat has a direct impact on the way your food is digested and assimilated. To get the most out of your food and support lit from within energy at the same time, find a space to eat where you'll be relaxed, grateful, and happy to savor the experience. Say a few words of gratitude or blessing over your meal (this both shifts energy and has physiological benefits that support digestion). And **remember that each time you bite or sip, you're literally eating energy, from both nutrients and feelings.** Enjoy!

Ready to begin your energetic day? Read on to welcome the energy of Sunrise.

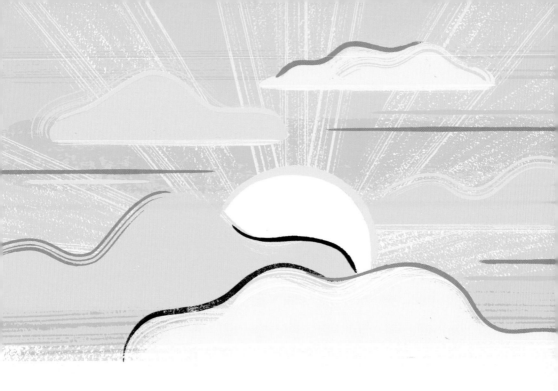

chapter two

Sunrise

Morning hours possess

undeniable magic.

The shades of light emitted as the sun peeks above the horizon feel otherworldly, pure, and exploding with possibility—altogether distinct from the retreating light at day's end. A sunrise is a promise of a fresh start; a real time, unfolding opportunity to live what you desire. Think of it as the springtime of your day. Even if you don't see yourself as a "morning person," there's so much that those early hours of the day have to offer your energy as a whole. Morning—and the energy you take from the morning hours—set the tone for your entire day, which then becomes a foundational element of your *life*! I believe that this part of the day holds the weightiest influence over your energy and your daily experience as a whole. At sunrise, you set the day's experience into motion. Are you ready to harness the beautifying, healing power of this moment? Let's start with your first action each morning: awakening.

Morning may be a time when your mind and body spring into action. Planning, preparing, and setting intentions for the hours to come are all key sunrise energy practices, but don't jump headfirst into the day without soaking in the significance of what may be the most important energetic opportunity of the 24-hour cycle: the moment you open your eyes. To change the energy of your morning, start by shifting how you awaken. Practice making your early morning moments look something like this gentle awakening sequence: Your mind slowly comes to focus; your eyes blink open. A new day stretches out before you. From exactly where you lie, become aware of your body by placing a hand on your abdomen while breathing in and out, feeling your core rise and fall. Gently extend your limbs a few inches, and point and flex your hands and feet, stretching your muscles. Observe yourself living, breathing, and deeply relaxed, and feel the goodness of this moment, wherever and whatever you are today. In a hyperconnected, fast-paced world, it's incredibly luxurious to slow down the act of rising and enter the day as if it were your first awakening. Let yourself savor that wakeup moment, whether it's fifteen seconds or five minutes.

Note: As you progress through this book, you may identify energetic shifts that you'd like to make in your daily routine. I've found that changing the pattern of your mornings can be a major catalyst for energetic shifts later in your day. As you use this book to guide your own morning routine, you may want to circle back to this chapter a few times, to allow yourself to continually adjust your goals and morning habits to spark change all day long.

SUNRISE ENERGY THEMES

beginning · preparing · awakening · envisioning · goal-setting · grooming · dressing · activating · centering

REFLECT ON YOUR SUNRISE ENERGY

What's the first thing I do when I awaken?

What's my energy like in the morning hours?

What are the biggest influences on my energy in the morning?

What interactions do I have, and what am I taking in early in the morning? News? E-mails? Conversations?

How does my morning routine prepare me for the day I hope to have?

Nature's Energy: Sun and Air

First thing in the morning, I love feeling the energy that comes from connection to the natural elements of the sun and the air. These elements are opening, expanding, giving of life and breath. Depending on the season and the hour that you rise, natural light may or may not greet you when you open your eyes. But a fresh breath of outside air is always there, on the other side of the window pane, a palpable connection to nature and the outdoors. Make it a part of your morning wakeup ritual to stop and throw open your window, step out onto your doorstep or fire escape, inhale deeply and feel the outside air on your face, whether it's

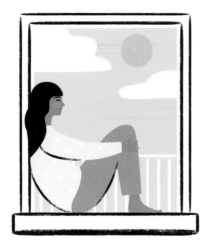

frosty or humid, breezy or still. You've just made your day's first energetic connection to nature.

When the sun has risen, spend some time in its morning rays to allow your body to soak up its solar energy and feel its balancing, recharging power. Regardless of season, the sun remains a vastly undervalued and often villainized source of healing energy. Morning sun specifically has a higher ratio of infrared light to UV radiation, and thus less potential to cause damage to the body and the skin. That extraordinary morning light enables the body to produce the antioxidant hormone melatonin, which plays a huge role in repair, regeneration, and overall antiaging in the body. Melatonin has 200 percent more antioxidant power than the celebrated skin protector vitamin E, and may be even more potent than the body's so-called master antioxidant, glutathione. Melatonin lowers inflammation, supports hormone balance, immunity, and adrenal function, and has even been shown in animal studies to extend life span. Our bodies synthesize melatonin in several ways, including through our retinas when we're exposed to morning light. Ten minutes of sunlight exposure first thing in the morning, every morning, will help you better synthesize melatonin and maintain healthy circadian rhythm—the daily, 24-hour cycle of our bodily functions, affecting everything from digestion, metabolism, aging, and immune function to temperature regulation, sleep, and alertness. Circadian rhythm is influenced by our exposure to light, dark, and temperature, so smart sun exposure is one of its most powerful cues. To get your morning sun, you might sip a smoothie while sitting in a sunny window, listen to a guided meditation outside, or take your morning movement outdoors. Even under a clouded sky, you'll be connected to that valuable light. Throughout the day, take periodic moments to connect to the sun (in moderation, of course), which boosts the availability of serotonin in your brain, lowers blood pressure, stimulates endorphin production (providing a mood boost), and activates parts of your immune system, in addition to enhancing energy. It's one mighty external energy source that's available to you every day.

RISING TO A CHALLENGE

When facing a challenge or struggle in your day or your daily life, your wakeup time can feel less than the power hour you want it to be. Instead of hope and possibility, the start of a new day can present an enormous obstacle laid out before you that brings anxiety, fear, or overwhelm. If you're feeling this way in the morning, I believe that the energy shifts in this chapter will help you feel more empowered and capable in the morning hours, or the early days of your challenge, as you accept that call to rise.

Use these habits to build your energy when you have something big to tackle:

* Start small. What's the very first step toward your goal?

* Wear a reminder of your commitment and power.

* Give yourself at least one specific thing to look forward to in the day ahead.

* Create and recite a mantra—make it your phone background or a periodic calendar reminder.

* Visualize the most positive outcome, over and over again!

* Rest and reward yourself each step of the way.

Top Sunrise Energy Drains

✳ **Reaching for your phone before you've taken time to awaken consciously**

✳ **Feeling that you are late or pressed for time from the minute you rise**

✳ **Failing to prep or think through essential parts of your routine the night before**

✳ **Viewing or reading upsetting news media as your first input of the day**

✳ **Jumping into your day without an intentional start**

✳ **Carrying yesterday's anger, worries, or fears into the new day**

SUNRISE ENERGY INFLUENCERS

I am endlessly captivated by the promise of the sunrise: the blank slate, the gift of another day, the new light that lets you see the same old things with fresh eyes. Sunrise is *your* moment to rise, and to raise your energy to increase the potential of the days and months ahead. **Your morning routine is incredibly powerful because it allows you to consciously step into your chosen energy for this day.** In this sunrise moment, your energy is particularly influenced by your mind, by your movements, and by the way you prepare the four facets of your energy—body, mind, emotions, and spirit—for the day. In this section, we'll look closely at these energy influencers, helping you to recognize their power to ignite your own inner light and transform the day that lies before you.

MORNING MESSAGING:
THE ENERGY OF YOUR MINDSET

Your most important sunrise opportunity comes from your conscious mind. Do you recall what your first conscious thought was this morning? That initial thought is quite telling—it often reflects where your mind has been in its deep state of rest, as well as the default mindset that you could project onto pretty much everyone and everything you encounter today. A negative state of mind, like fear, worry, or jealousy, in the morning produces an unwelcome effect on your energy that can easily grow and spiral out of control over the course of the day. If your first conscious thought is related to worry, stress, or dread, you've already begun a pattern of dim energy, perhaps based solely in your mind, that's certain to impact your behavior and your choices in the hours ahead.

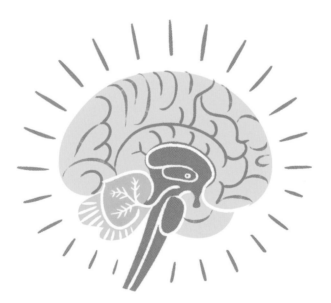

Negative thoughts have been found to create physical inflammation in the body by stimulating the production of pro-inflammatory cytokines. To give your inner light a powerful burst of bright energy instead, aim to make your first thoughts ones of possibility, joy, love, contentment, and gratitude. **Your body "hears" and responds to your mind energetically, giving even your unspoken thoughts, affirmations, and intentions power that can't be overstated.** In fact, your state of mind creates an energetic effect that sweeps over every cell in your body, producing dramatic changes in your personal energy. In addition to inflammation, your thoughts alone can shift physical aspects of the body, such as heart rate, blood pressure, body temperature, rate of breathing, digestion, perspiration, and muscle tension.

As you wake, your body emerges from a state of deep healing, resetting, and balancing, and transitions back to what's likely to be a demanding, high-output portion of your day. The way that process happens for you also has serious bearing on the energy you'll carry. The transition period from sleep to wake is one that I imagine to be a little like a rebirth—entering the conscious world again, for what could be a brand-new experience; it's really up to you. With a little intention and practice, you can direct that reentry with every sunrise.

What's the best way to harness the energetic possibility of the sunrise? First, observe. Spend just a few minutes visualizing the act of waking up in your body and reconnecting to your alert consciousness as if you're seeing it from above. What are the patterns that you see happening as you awaken and rise each day? What distractions or challenges do you face? Where can you make shifts to protect your body's transitional moments and set yourself on your desired energetic path for the day? You might take a morning or two just to notice what happens in you and around you at wakeup time, thinking about what works for you, and what doesn't support the energy you'd like to feel as you awaken. What are you feeling, and what are your needs? Practice creating a wakeup routine that lets you savor that act of waking up, rather than rushing through it. You may find that it helps to spend a portion of your morning wakeup alone, building your energy for the day ahead consciously and without interruption—a challenge for many of us, including myself! Although morning isn't always about you (kids, pets, partners, relatives, friends, or work likely make considerable demands on your morning time), you'll have better control of your energy all day if you can take a few minutes to connect to the way you'd like to feel during the day ahead. (And promise me that you'll at least *occasionally* set aside a morning that's completely yours)!

Change Your Brain

No matter what's unfolding in your life today, the way you perceive and react to it is up to you. If you find that you've developed morning mental patterns that you'd like to change, begin the adjustment process now. Know that you can undo whatever daily habits you've developed as long as you make the effort. Your brain possesses an astonishing quality called neuroplasticity that gives you the potential to rewire your default responses, thoughts, and habits.

Here's one way to start that rewiring process in your brain to default to positivity, gratitude, and joy in the morning: As you open your eyes and regain alertness after sleep, concentrate first on a positive feeling. Maybe you're warm and comfortable in your sheets, the rays of sun entering your bedroom look soft and welcoming, or you notice that you're breathing calmly and effortlessly. Right where you lie, without moving or fast-forwarding into your day, there is good here. When you start by finding that moment of good, it's easier to transition into gratitude and possibility in whatever lies ahead. If you find negative thoughts arising (my back hurts, I have so much to do today, it's Monday and it's raining), catch them (hold on there—gotcha), name them (okay, this is my fear talking), and then dismiss them—go ahead and picture yourself swatting them out of the way or rubbing them away with an eraser. Replace each tossed-out thought with a brighter thought or truth, crowding out any dim energy that creeps in out of habit. And as you do, really let yourself *feel* this gratitude and moment of happiness. As it's happening, if you are consciously aware that you feel happy and grateful, the mental and physical effects become even more pro-found. What you pay attention to truly shapes your reality. Let the pleasure and possibility of the moment sink in—hold that thought, literally!

How does that happiness or contentment or safety feel in your body? Take a moment to picture the neurons and pathways in your brain being activated and lighting up in new and stronger patterns of happiness. In the early days of this routine, you're priming the process; faking it until you make it, just as smiling has been shown to create happiness by urging your brain to generate positive emotions. But the more you practice, the greater the gratitude muscle that develops, and the more you become effortlessly swept up in a new mental pattern that lights you up.

Just as your existing defaults likely took months or years to form, the rewiring process won't happen overnight. (Remember the negativity bias on page 27?) So, start reinforcing the mental patterns you want today. It's excit-ing how quickly a new routine forms—some research says 66 days while oth-ers point to 21 days (or even less!) for a new habit to become automatic. Like the food on your plate and the clothes that you wear (more on that ahead), your experience and timeline of change will depend most on your individual body; but know that it's well within your power to make a massive shift in your thought patterns.

When you make your morning brain workout one of gratitude—even (and especially) on challenging days—you also give an incredible boost to your per-sonal energy. Gratitude is one of the most profound keys to your happiness, resilience, and inner light. The magic lies in your perspective. In the morning, gratitude can be as simple as thinking or saying aloud, "Thank you for the gift of a new day to experience here on Earth." Putting into place a ritual of gratitude creates a default direction for your energy in those early morning moments as you regain your conscious thoughts. Using gratitude, you ensure that your mind doesn't jump immediately into stresses or to-dos and instead gets a reminder to look around and be present for good things.

Gratitude has been shown to increase happiness, reduce depression, strengthen mental resilience and self-esteem, improve sleep and self-care habits, and stimulate empathy toward others, among its many profound benefits. And if you're not feeling especially grateful for anything at the moment, look around you and express gratitude for simple, seemingly insignificant stuff: a paint color that you like on the wall, the yummy-smelling lip balm on your bedside table, or the pet that's waking you from sleep because he wants to be fed. If you enjoy the act of writing, reach over to your bedside table for a notebook and pen (yes, keep them there!) and make a list of the things that are lighting up your gratitude pathways this morning. Resist the urge to react, and be reactive, in this moment. If you truly can't sit quietly for a few minutes (say you have a child crying or a bus to catch), take a second to let one positive thought sink in and then return to your gratitude and intentional awakening later in your day.

Shifting Your Subconscious

Have you ever awoken and not immediately remembered where you were? As your mind transitions from sleep to wake, there are often a few moments where your consciousness is a bit fuzzy. Those are the transitional moments when your brain waves are shifting, and they're some of the best times to access your subconscious mind to change mental patterns. What's so special about your subconscious? It's estimated that your conscious mind, while itself a powerful entity, controls only about 5 percent of your cognitive activity. Your subconscious—the brain activity of which you don't have awareness—controls the other 95 percent. I find it incredibly exciting that, with practice, you can alter and influence your subconscious, to ensure that it serves you as an asset toward reaching and maintaining the energy that you desire.

First thing in the morning, your brain is just emerging from sleep, making it easier to slip into a relaxed state of alpha brain waves—the brain state that you reach when you daydream or practice a light meditation—and more readily affect your subconscious mind. This is one of the reasons a mantra can be such a powerful force for change during meditation, a time when you also enter an alpha or theta (even deeper) brain wave state. While you're becoming conscious yet still in a relaxed state, you're much better able to visualize, imagine, concentrate, and reprogram your thoughts.

This is an ideal time to incorporate an affirmation—a definitive statement or assertion that something is true—that will help steer your subconscious toward a positive mindset or goal. Create your own affirmation and repeat it throughout the day, either in your mind or aloud. With continued repetition, your subconscious mind begins to reflexively respond as if your affirmation is true. I find simple affirmations to be the easiest to remember and repeat often. Try starting yours with the words "I am." The statement "I am calm, I am strong, I am well" was one that I repeated over and over during my healing process, often in the relaxed moments just after waking. I also encourage you to speak your affirmations out loud sometimes—a practice that I find to be especially helpful. When you speak words aloud, you strongly reinforce their message by creating memories of hearing your statements in addition to your thoughts of them.

Another fascinating tool that allows you to shift your subconscious at any time of day is visualization. As the name implies, during visualization you picture or visualize your desired feeling or outcome. Your subconscious mind, dominant as it may be, can't tell the difference between reality and imagination, especially when you create a specific mental picture or imagined experience and allow yourself to feel its associated emotions. In deceiving your subconscious in this way, you can give your mind positive images and experiences to focus on again and again. You'll practice this ahead. Visualization is best done in a relaxed state, and you can even use brain-training tools, like binaural beats audio (see page 171), to bring your brain into a relaxed alpha or theta state while you visualize.

These mindset tools can create major shifts in your body and your life, especially if you're consistent about practicing them. Incorporating them into your morning routine is one way to ensure that you take advantage of them daily. Above all, remember that your body hears your thoughts and responds to them. If you haven't yet connected your thoughts to your reality, this may be one of your biggest takeaways from this book. Curbing complaining and negative self-talk (and replacing them with bright energy via thoughts, affirmations, and visualization) breaks a self-destructive habit and can completely change your reality and the energy of your body. New, positive mental patterns unleash untold amounts of confidence and self-esteem that were only being withheld from you by your mind. When you don't believe you're worthy of all of the beauty, health, happiness, and joy that any given day can hold, you can keep yourself from experiencing it. If you have fallen into the habit of complaints and negative self-talk, you can get so much closer to feeling lit from within just by eliminating these perpetual energy drains. Your mind is wildly powerful and, with practice, you'll make it one of your most supportive energy tools.

My biggest mindset energy shift came when:
I stopped jumping out of bed before I had time to say a morning prayer, express gratitude, and get clear on my daily intention.

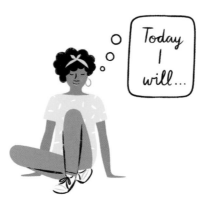

MIND ENERGY IN PRACTICE:
MORNING INTENTION-SETTING

Once you begin to brighten your morning mindset, you'll likely feel expanded possibility in your life, as you create a brain state that opens you to opportunity and exploration. But with all of that possibility, where will you choose to go? And what will you choose to do? Morning brings another opportunity to direct your day's journey by getting clear on your biggest dreams, goals, and desires—the intentions you'd like to bring to fruition. An intention-setting ritual is an opportunity to use your thoughts, words, and mindset to focus yourself ahead of the day and actively guide the path of your life. It's a seed that, when planted in your mind, becomes more likely to grow and flourish.

To create such a ritual in your morning, set aside a few moments to focus on your desired outcome for the day. Personally, it helps me to start with general hopes and then become more specific, like this:

I sit or lie comfortably and breathe, ensuring that I'm taking long, slow, relaxed breaths. When my mind is free of distractions, I like to first express gratitude for a new day that brings so much potential. A mindset of gratitude is an ideal energetic state before intention-setting begins; it opens you to possibility. Then, I express my willingness to use this day in my life for a larger purpose, perhaps a purpose of which I haven't even conceived. I think and/or speak the intention that I be guided to do the things, meet the people, and speak the words that will keep me on the path of healing, beauty, and light, for myself and others, across this day. If I have a specific desired outcome, I take a few minutes to visualize it with clarity and specificity, remembering to allow myself to experience all the good feelings that accompany that event (joy of a success, peace from resolution of a problem, a positive breakthrough in a creative project, etc.).

You might choose to write down your intentions for your day in a journal, in your phone, or in a place where you can display them and think of them often. You might also find or create a special place that feels conducive to intention-setting: a light-filled corner, a comfy chair, a backyard spot where you can dig your toes into the grass. Any place that helps the moment to feel more significant, sacred, and filled with bright energy is perfect. Can you also set intentions while commuting on a crowded subway? Totally. When in doubt, keep your intentions focused on the short term. Give your mind lots of clear examples of how this goal could come about, a practice that lets your mind know that your desires are possible. Continue to ingrain this with your thoughts across your day, and return tomorrow for another intention-filled start.

⇒ Energy Booster ⇐

To make your intention reality, to become the person you want to be, to get to your goal or destination, start thinking of yourself as if you're already there. Don't get stuck waiting to feel 100 percent, to lose 5 more pounds, or to get the job you want—seize the power of now. When you do, you'll feel a spark of energy that helps you take a major leap toward your goal, even as you trick your body and mind to consistently move in the direction of that reality.

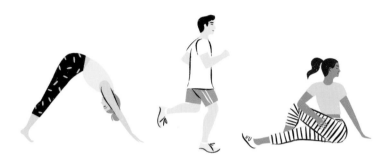

GET PHYSICAL:
THE ENERGY OF MOVEMENT

To feel your energy shift in real time, take a moment right now to stand up and move your body. Stretch toward the sky and feel expansive; sway side to side and feel soothed; jump in place a dozen times and feel enthusiastic; do a set of push-ups and feel dominant. There are about as many ways to move your body as there are bodies in the world. With movement, as with nutrition, I truly believe that the best form for you is unique to your body. Also as with nutrition, that ideal movement may change based on any number of variables: the season, your hormonal cycles, your age, the weather, your mood, or your mindset. However you choose to move your body, know that **movement is vital not only for strength and fitness, but for emotional health, freedom, confidence, and creation of the energy state you desire.** Moving your body helps circulate energy and nutrition, rev up detox processes, strengthen the immune system, and calm anxiety and reactivity.

When I think about morning awakening after a night of rest, I imagine a spark going off within me, not far off from the visual of the sunrise breaking through a dark sky. You feel that spark in your mind as you prepare to flow through your morning routine and tackle the day's plans. And you feel it in your body, where it becomes the energy that springs you into action, creating movement. Although movement is a tool to employ throughout the day, it's especially powerful in the morning hours, when it supports your energy as you awaken. Make time for movement, every single morning? Before you worry that you'll have to get up earlier, skip breakfast, or overhaul your current schedule to fit it in, let me clarify: movement need not mean a 3-mile run, 30 minutes of circuit training, or even breaking a sweat. I define movement as literally moving your body in any way you so choose to achieve the energetic shift you desire. Exercise is a type of movement, but it's only one way to move. Others are bending, twisting, and playing.

Make your movement choices intuitive, freeing, and joyful, based on your needs. What energetic result do you wish to yield today? Seek out types of movement that enable you to sink into and extend the feel of your desired energetic state. If you typically rush through a spinning session so you can then hop in the shower, shoot out the door, and make it to the office on time, you may be doing everything that you think you *should* do, yet coming up short energetically. To feel more balanced and tranquil, you may want to shorten the intense portion of your workout but take extra time to warm up and cool down. If simple stretches are not delivering the focus and momentum you need in the morning, add more dynamic movements that get your heart pumping, or go for a brisk jog that can help you release energy or emotions you don't want to bring into the new day.

To more fully experience an energy shift from movement, I encourage you to move without measure. Forget the numbers. Put away the clocks and timers. How often do you check the time while you're working out? How many of your fitness goals are related to time, distance, calories burned, repetitions, or another numerical measure of success? My analytical mind sets and achieves goals by numbers as much as anyone, but I've since learned how much that approach clouds my energetic experience of movement—an end goal I don't want to lose sight of. For the purpose of energy exploration, let the numbers go today. Maybe you set an alarm so you don't lose complete track of time and miss your next commitment. But let go of all other measures of time and distance, and just move.

If you had to move to achieve the energy state you wanted today, how would you do it? Would you put on your favorite song and jump, sway, spin, reach, etc. until you felt amazing? Would you lace up your sneakers and run as fast as you could until you'd released everything that had been weighing you down? Would you call a friend and hike through a forest until you reached a site that conveyed the peace you're seeking this morning? While you're at it, pay attention to your movement sweet spot. Too much exertion can run us dry, while too little can trap energy within our bodies that negatively affects each of our four energy facets. Can you push yourself until you feel energy flow, yet stop before overdoing it? There's your energetic sweet spot.

Move All Day

Movement is so powerful and so instant an energy-shifter that you should absolutely be employing it again and again throughout your day. Sunrise brings your first opportunity, and it's a powerful one, promising to inform your energy all day long. But what about mid-morning, after sitting at your desk for a few hours? (Just as movement can create energy, sitting for hours can sap it away). Or during an afternoon slump? How about right before bed? For your most consistent energy, practice intermittent movement breaks throughout the day, every 90 to 120 minutes, giving yourself 5 to 10 minutes to move each time (for more on why these breaks support your energy, see page 110). This way, 10 minutes of movement quickly becomes 30, 40, 60, or more, spread evenly and consistently across your day. Incidentally, just 10 minutes of gentle movement has been shown to increase activity in the areas of your brain linked to memory processing and storage; a little break to move can help you process and digest what's going on in your day.

Another important gift of movement throughout your day is the opportunity to release. As the day wears on, periodic movement breaks help stimulate energy flow and release energy that weighs you down or affects your focus (read more about the energy of release on page 206). Make it a goal to release stuck energy (you may feel this in the form of tension, distraction, stress, or other emotion) little by little throughout the day.

I find it fascinating that movement creates energy in part by challenging and stressing the body, an unlikely catalyst for repair and strengthening that results in an overall health and healing boost. Movement stimulates the flow of lymph, the waste-removing fluid that is so important to detox and whole-body health. It also increases blood flow to tissues and releases chemicals that support immune function, healing, and good moods (think: endorphins, dopamine, serotonin), which in turn affect the radiance of your skin.

Of course, more is not always more—too much, too vigorous exercise day after day can become a stressor for your body's hormonal balance, especially in combination with a high-stress life. If this sounds like you, incorporate more forms of movement that lower the stress hormone cortisol and leave you feeling restored rather than depleted. Think: walking, yoga, and—if you're looking for something unexplored that's deeply connected to energy—consider Qigong. This five-thousand-year-old healing practice (its name translates to "the exercise of life energy") resets posture, breath, and mindset in support of health, joy, and appreciation of beauty in the present moment. It's accessible to all skill levels and can be done in a small space (e.g., a hotel room while traveling or your office at work).

Regardless of the movement you choose, it helps to be confident of its value for your four energy facets. One interesting study found that, among two groups who performed the same activities, there were significantly greater health gains (including markers like weight loss, reduced blood pressure, and improved BMI) in the group that was told all about the health benefits of their activities before performing them. So, get your mind involved. You might even pepper your next workout with fitness affirmations, such as "I am getting stronger with every repetition," or "I am firing up my mitochondria with each step," or "I'm moving toward bright energy with every breath." Combine your mindset energy with movement energy to help yourself shine even brighter.

My biggest movement energy shift came when:
I based my daily movement choices on the way they made me feel,
rather than numerical goals.

MOVEMENT ENERGY IN PRACTICE:
SUN SALUTATION

A morning sun salutation (the name given to a series of yoga poses practiced in a continuous sequence) is a lovely way to awaken your body and activate a feeling of grounding, calming, and opening through flowing movement. It's modifiable for all skill and strength levels. If you want to take the opportunity to move in the morning but you're short on time, this practice is particularly ideal for you. Its pose sequence stretches and gently activates muscles, increases circulation and lymph flow, allows for deep, cleansing breaths, and connects your mind to the power of the sun all within a few minutes. It feels like a physical manifestation of my morning gratitude practice, as I let my movements express my appreciation for the sun, which fuels another day of light, energy, and life on Earth.

Ready to begin? You can vary this basic sun salutation to suit your body and your favorite yoga poses. It's yet another way you can switch up your movement as needed. I like to stand near a window where I can see the sky or feel a breeze of outside air to connect to nature during this practice.

Stand with your feet flat on the ground, shoulder width apart, and feel your soles firmly rooted to the ground.

Place your hands together at your chest, touching the area of your heart.

Inhaling slowly and deeply, stretch your arms toward the sky. Really stretch, as far as it feels good to you, experiencing your lungs expanding and opening up space in your abdomen.

When you're ready to exhale, fold forward at the waist and let your torso hang down, stretching toward your feet and exhaling completely. The back stretch here is my favorite!

Raise your arms and inhale again as you move down onto one bended knee.

As you exhale, fold forward, plant your hands on the ground and push back into downward dog pose, then push forward until you are flat on the ground with your stomach touching the floor in a low plank.

Push your arms and chest up into cobra pose as you inhale and stretch your core and chest.

Push back into downward dog pose as you exhale.

Walk your arms back until you're standing in a forward bend, then begin the sequence again by standing upright and stretching your arms to the sky as you inhale.

Fold down to touch your toes as you exhale deeply.

Raise your arms and inhale again as you move down onto one bended knee (this time, choose the opposite knee to bend).

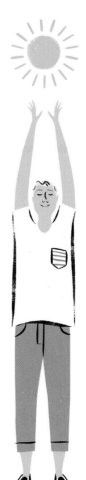

Fold forward into downward dog pose as you exhale, then push forward until you are flat on the ground with your stomach touching the floor.

Push your arms and chest up into cobra pose as you inhale and stretch your core and chest.

Push back into downward dog pose as you exhale.

Walk your arms back until you're standing in a forward bend.

Inhale once more as you return upright, stretching your arms to the sky and finishing with your hands together at your chest, breathing normally.

You can practice this sequence several times in succession, at a pace you prefer, making it slow and methodical or fast and brisk. I find that I can move through it several times almost without thinking, which gives me the time to continue to awaken gently. If you're not able to achieve these poses because of an injury or health issue, create your own sequence that centers on stretching and breathing in a way that feels good to you. And if you'd like to move onto something more dynamic, follow with a few minutes of cardio or strength training (classic push-ups build more vigorous energy when you're short on time!). Practice this sequence outdoors, standing barefoot on grass, dirt, or sand, for an extra challenge that lets you connect to the earth and the energy of the sun and air at sunrise.

⇒ Energy Booster ⇐

The body and brain are complex, but building bright energy within them doesn't have to be. Next time you're moving outdoors, focus your mind and find bright energy around you using my "So Good" exercise. This ultra-simple practice is ideal on a walk or a run, or anytime your mind tends to wander to worries or stress. As you move, look around you (or within you, for that matter!) and find one thing that's "so good"—go ahead and use your own words if you like. Think, "That breeze blowing on my face is so good." Or "Those vibrant pink tulips are so good." Now feel the energy of your chosen focus; does the breeze soothe you, or are those tulips so vivid that you can't help but smile? As you focus on and really soak in that feeling, direct it to a place in your body—choose a place that needs to heal, if you have one, otherwise direct it to your heart—and feel it there. After you've taken in that feeling for a moment or two, find your next "so good" item and continue the process. This is one of my favorite ways to redirect my mind from worries or rumination, and it helps me appreciate the beautiful little things I'd otherwise overlook!

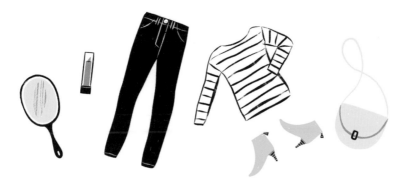

WELL BEGUN:
THE ENERGY OF PREPARATION

Morning is the time to put on your energy armor. You've already done so in your mindset and in your physical movements; now let's match those to your appearance. This could mean in color, meaningful objects, or accessories, your personal power uniform (you know, that one outfit that makes you feel unstoppable), or whatever articles speak to you in that moment. No single one is better than another, so pick what triggers a feeling of bright energy when you see it or put it on.

Preparing yourself for the day might be a steady, well-rehearsed routine, or a moment of serendipity and self-reflection that comes to you in each new day. While the decision of what to wear and how to prepare yourself may not feel so important at seven a.m., its consequence is clear every time you pass a mirror, catch your reflection in a pane of glass, or stand before another human. And that's not even counting all of the times you snap a selfie, if that's your thing. In every one of these instances, your appearance triggers an energy shift, consciously and subconsciously keeping you on track with the intentional decisions you make in this morning moment. Your appearance itself becomes an energetic possession that you carry with you until you change it. So, what energy, what persona, what characteristics will you turn on this morning as you prepare yourself?

I love the anecdote of Marilyn Monroe walking along Fifth Avenue in New York City, unnoticed among the crowds. To the amazement of her companion, she offered to "turn on" her movie-star persona, visibly changed her posture and step, and within minutes was thronged by fans. Think of the morning hours as the time for you to turn on your light, for yourself and for others, as you greet the day. The way you prepare yourself not only affects the energy that others perceive, it affects your own energy for the entire day. What are you preparing for today? Prepare for the good outcome, the stroke of luck, the serendipity, the blessing. When you prepare for it, you'll find it—and be ready to receive.

If I could give just one piece of advice for the energy of preparation, it would be: dress for the way you want to feel. You woke up with puffy eyes and a headache? Dress like you've never been in better health and you feel like a queen. Want to ace an exam? Skip the sweats and pull together a polished look. Nervous about a formal event? Choose the softest, most comforting fabrics in colors that make you feel confident and at ease. Don't make preparation an afterthought, because your morning choices will literally stay with you for hours—if not for the entire day. **The world is a visual place, and the way you prepare yourself makes a statement before you speak—exactly like your energy.** Remember that you're dressing for yourself and for your desire to shift your personal energy and experience for this entire day. If you're still on your journey (aren't we all?) to look a certain way, find your healthiest weight, feel more confident about your features, or get the job or promotion you want, prepare yourself as though you've already reached that goal. Prepare yourself in celebration of the absolute beauty that you possess here and now.

What about grooming? If preparation includes makeup and personal care products for you, as it does for most of us, I urge you to consider the long-term energetic effect of the products you apply to your body. Too many beauty formulas still compromise energy and health with ingredients that are harmful (and in particular disruptive of hormonal health) and unrecognizable to your body. Since you absorb the majority of the ingredients you apply to your skin, dosing yourself with these ingredients day after day places unneeded stress on your body—a certain influence on your energy as well.

The relieving news is that swapping potentially toxic beauty formulas for healthier products quickly changes the landscape of your body. Study shows that within days after you stop exposure, levels of questionable ingredients like parabens, phthalates, chemical sunscreens, and antibacterial triclosan drop as these ingredients are removed from your body. No matter what your age or your profession, you can shift your own energy by choosing products with ingredients that support rather than diminish your health and energy. While you're scrutinizing your products, take a hard look at your current personal care routine and reflect on which of its aspects are truly helping you to feel your best, and which could be hiding your authentic self. Get rid of any outdated beliefs about the way you need to appear, for yourself or anyone else; these are instant ways to dim your energy. Let your beauty and energy shine through in a way that feels right to you, regardless of what anyone else chooses. Sometimes the energy and ideals of others unconsciously become our own over time; consider whether or not you need to shake those off and reconnect to yourself, which brings its own visible shift in your energy.

A note about our relationship with our physical body: there is deep beauty and health in feeling confidence, contentment, and love for what you see in the mirror; and for continually working to look your best, *if* you're motivated by self-love, pleasure, and wellness. I call the desire to look and live as your best self "healthy vanity," because of its benefits for mind and body. If you're working on your appearance to earn the admiration or approval of others, however, eventually you are almost certain to fall short. When it comes to your own unique beauty, let this book inspire you to light yourself up in ways that are first and foremost perceptible to you alone. I promise, there will still be shifts, both physical and energetic, that make others take notice. The impact you make with your energy is so much more profound and lasting than appearance alone.

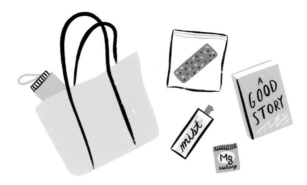

Prepare for the Energy You Want

Fail to plan, plan to fail, right? Energetic preparation also means planning for the day ahead. A preparation energy tip I love: pack a little something that will give you an instant energy shift later on in your day. It could be a Sesame Glow Bar (see page 95) to recharge you midmorning, a cooling aromatherapy face mist that you can use to spritz your skin after your commute, or the book you can't wait to pick up on your lunch break. If you have a long day ahead of you, it might even be a change of clothing or shoes to make sure your appearance matches the energy you want in whatever activities pop up. You'll never catch me without at least one little item that can influence my energy—or the energy of my son—when I'm out and about; a de-stressing essential oil roll-on and packets of my favorite magnesium drink are staples.

My biggest preparation energy shift came when:
I started dressing and grooming for the way I wanted to feel, even on the days that my health was the poorest.

PREPARATION ENERGY IN PRACTICE: DRESSING IN COLOR

Get calming vibes from your baby blue skirt? Or feel fired up whenever you wear red? It's not just rumor or your imagination—colors have their own energy and even their own *vibration*. While there's no single way to correctly interpret colors, you can use your wardrobe to experiment with the energy-shifting role that colors play in your life. Our perception of an object's color depends on how it reflects and absorbs light. Light is necessary to see the millions of colors (perhaps 7 to 10 million) that our eyes can distinguish. Each color has its own vibration, from violet (the color with the highest vibration and shortest wavelength, giving it a reputation for "high vibes" and an association with the crown chakra) in reverse rainbow order (remember your ROYGBIV?) down to red, which has the lowest vibration and longest wavelength, making it a more grounding hue that is associated with the root chakra.

The following are some of the popular interpretations of color meaning and energy, including their corresponding chakras where they apply (flip back to page 34 for more on chakras). This, of course, depends on the shade of each particular color; fuchsia pink conveys much more intensity than soft rose, for example. How many of these interpretations align with your own?

※ **RED:** *passion, strength, intensity, power, love//root chakra*

※ **ORANGE:** *stimulation, spiritedness//sacral chakra*

※ **YELLOW:** *optimism, joy, mental clarity//solar plexus chakra*

※ **GREEN:** *healing, balance, fertility, harmony//heart chakra*

※ **BLUE:** *calm, wisdom, serenity//throat chakra*

※ **PURPLE/VIOLET:** *royalty, creativity//crown chakra*

PINK: *femininity, compassion, youth, romance*

WHITE: *purity, goodness*

BROWN: *earthiness, groundedness, stability*

BLACK: *mystery, formality, elegance, power, intelligence*

GRAY: *formality, neutrality, detachment*

Think about your own relationship with the color in your wardrobe. Which colors feature most prominently in your closet? Consider your shoes and accessories as well as clothing.

Which colors make you happiest?

Which colors help you feel the energetic state you choose for yourself today?

Which colors look best on your unique skin, hair, and eye coloring?

Which colors are missing entirely?

Using your answers to these questions, choose to wear more of the colors that support the energy of your happiness, or the other specific energetic state you want to bring in to your life.

⇒ Energy Booster ⇐

Take a selfie each day this week, before you leave the house. What feelings do you get when you look back at this series of photographs at the end of the week? What do these pictures and the way you prepare yourself, convey about your personal energy?

LAUREL'S SUNRISE

NAME: Laurel Shaffer

WHAT TO KNOW ABOUT ME:
I am a skincare product formulator who connects people to nature through beauty rituals.

THE SUNRISE HOURS OF MY DAY ARE USUALLY:
Slow and thoughtful.

MY ESSENTIALS FOR THE BEST SUNRISE ENERGY:
Kundalini and meditation, whole plant products, and cuddling with my dogs.

FAVORITE WAY TO FUEL MY BODY DURING SUNRISE HOURS:
I do my best to make time for 15 minutes of kundalini yoga warmups, followed by 15 minutes of meditation. This practice of greeting my body, mind, and spirit in the early morning keeps me focused and calm throughout the busy day ahead.

SUNRISE ENERGY INFLUENCERS AFFECT MY PERSONAL ENERGY MOST IN THE AREA OF:
Preparation. Both my own skincare products and my favorite line of flower essences play a large role in my mornings. I use flower essences before and after morning meditation. My morning skincare ritual is never the same; I reach for the products that contain whatever plants call to me. This process of intuitively selecting products and then mindfully experiencing them can be like another meditation in itself. I'm always grateful that these plants not only bolster the health of my skin, but also offer energetic support to me at the start of each day.

More Ways to Feel the Energy of Sunrise

✳ Get up and watch the sun rise at least once a year to remember its transformative power.

✳ Awaken in the dark and practice your preferred morning exercise by candlelight as the sky shifts to light.

✳ Create your perfect morning beverage, ideally one that combines hydration, antioxidants, and detox support. Try the Green Beauty Broth recipe on page 92 for one of my personal favorites.

✳ Get up with a sunrise wakeup lamp in the darker months so that your body can experience the gentle light shift of a sunrise at your preferred wakeup time. You can also use it to create a natural sundown at bedtime!

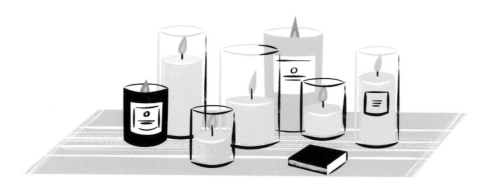

RECIPES TO NOURISH YOUR SUNRISE ENERGY

Morning is the time to refuel after hours of rest, and it's an ideal opportunity to choose foods that transfer their energetic capacity to your body when you eat them. Your breakfast choices, like your morning thoughts and rituals, set the tone for your energy and your physical performance over the rest of the day. What should you look for in your morning meal? The best sunrise energy foods deliver rehydration and sustaining fuel that support blood sugar stability; stimulate the senses to further the awakening process in your body; and offer a store of antioxidant phytochemicals that your body can draw from all day, in support of looking and feeling your best. I remind my readers and clients to choose meals with the essential trio of healthy fats, clean protein, and abundant fresh produce to support optimal skin health, hormone balance, their health-iest weight, and to ensure that they feel full and satisfied rather than hungry and snacky. Ahead are some of my favorite recipes that provide these sunrise essentials. Prepare them and savor them across the morning hours to fuel each fresh start.

Ideal foods for sunrise energy:
healthy fats like nut butter, avocado, and coconut; clean protein, like pastured eggs, hempseeds, or collagen; nutrient-dense greens and herbs; water-rich fruit.

Sunday Morning Ginger-Apple Fritters with Raw Honey Glaze

I love Sunday morning energy—calm, slow, indulgent. Take some extra time to peel apples, grate aromatic ginger, and savor the process of making these addictive (yet protein-packed) bites.

MAKES 20 FRITTERS

Coconut oil, for pan

1 cup/110 g blanched almond flour

1 cup/140 g gluten-free flour blend (I like Bob's Red Mill 1-to-1)

¼ cup/30 g arrowroot starch

2 teaspoons baking powder

½ teaspoon baking soda

Scant ½ teaspoon unrefined salt

¾ cup/200 ml unsweetened nondairy milk

1 teaspoon apple cider vinegar

2 tablespoons/30 ml pure maple syrup

1 (½-inch/13mm) piece fresh ginger, scrubbed and grated with a Micro-plane grater or zester

1½ cups/200 g peeled and diced organic apple (about 1½ apples)

GLAZE

¾ cup/90 g raw cashews

1 tablespoon raw honey

5 tablespoons/80 ml water

⅛ teaspoon almond extract

Preheat the oven to 375°F/190°C. Grease a mini muffin pan with the coconut oil.

In a large bowl, combine the flours, arrowroot, baking powder, baking soda, and salt. In a smaller bowl, whisk together the milk, vinegar, and maple syrup. Pour the wet ingredients into the dry, and fold in the ginger and apple. Fill each prepared muffin well until slightly mounded with batter. Bake for 20 minutes, or until golden. Repeat with remaining batter.

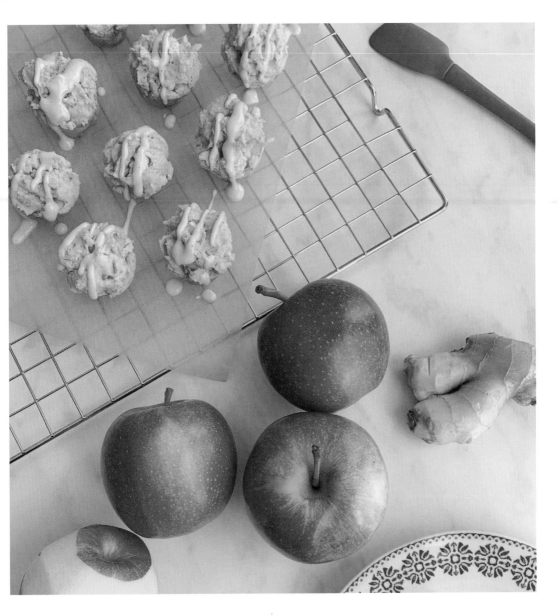

While the fritters bake, combine the glaze ingredients in a high-powered blender and process until smooth, scraping down the sides if needed. Remove the fritters from the oven, let cool slightly, and serve drizzled with the raw honey glaze.

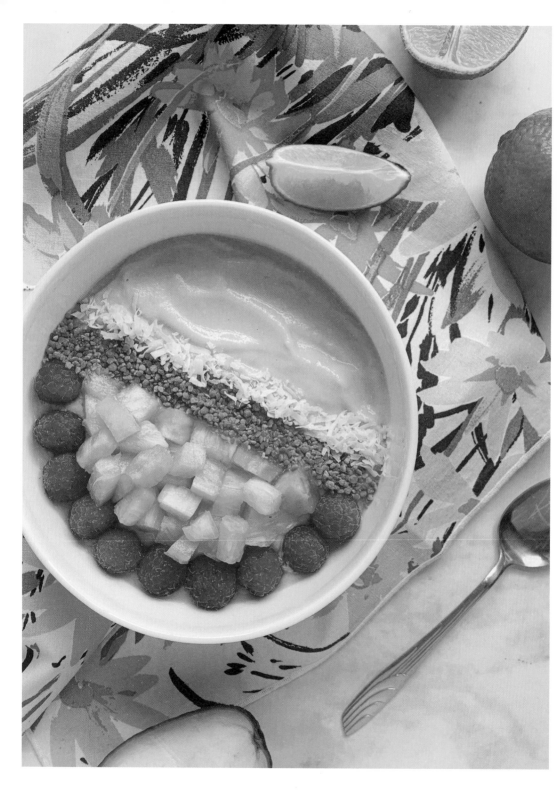

Vacation Vibes Avocado Smoothie Bowl

Island-inspired breakfast ingredients brighten my energy, even on a cloudy day. This smoothie bowl will sustain you for hours, thanks to its combination of healthy fats, collagen protein, and nutrient-dense veggies.

SERVES 1

½ ripe avocado, pitted and peeled

Juice of 1 lime

½ cup/65 g frozen cauliflower

¾ cup/120 g fresh or frozen pineapple chunks

¾ cup/200 ml unsweetened nondairy milk (coconut tastes best here)

1 tablespoon unsweetened shredded coconut, plus more for topping

1 serving collagen powder (I like Vital Proteins Marine Collagen Peptides)

½ teaspoon maca powder

Bee pollen, fresh fruit, and/or raw nuts and seeds for topping (optional)

In a high-powered blender, combine the avocado, lime juice, cauliflower, pineapple, and milk until smooth. Add the coconut, collagen, and maca and blend to incorporate. Transfer to a bowl and top with additional shredded coconut, bee pollen, fruit, nuts, and seeds, if desired. Serve immediately.

Grounding Sunrise Omelet

This recipe makes a perfect power breakfast to build physical energy for the day—and it easily scales to serve a crowd. I love its vivid sunrise colors—from bright yellow pastured yolks to vibrant carrots—that help awaken my senses in the early morning hours.

SERVES 1

2 teaspoons unsalted grass-fed organic butter or ghee

Heaping ¼ cup/50 g shredded organic carrot

2 large mushrooms (I like shiitake), stems removed, chopped

2 large pastured eggs, beaten

Unrefined salt

Ground black pepper

Small handful of roughly chopped carrot tops and other assorted greens

In a nonstick skillet, melt the butter over medium heat and sauté the shredded carrot and mushrooms until the mushrooms reduce slightly, about 3 minutes. Pour the beaten eggs over the vegetables, season with salt and pepper, and cook over low heat until the omelet reaches your desired doneness. Fold the omelet, remove it from the pan, and serve alongside fresh greens.

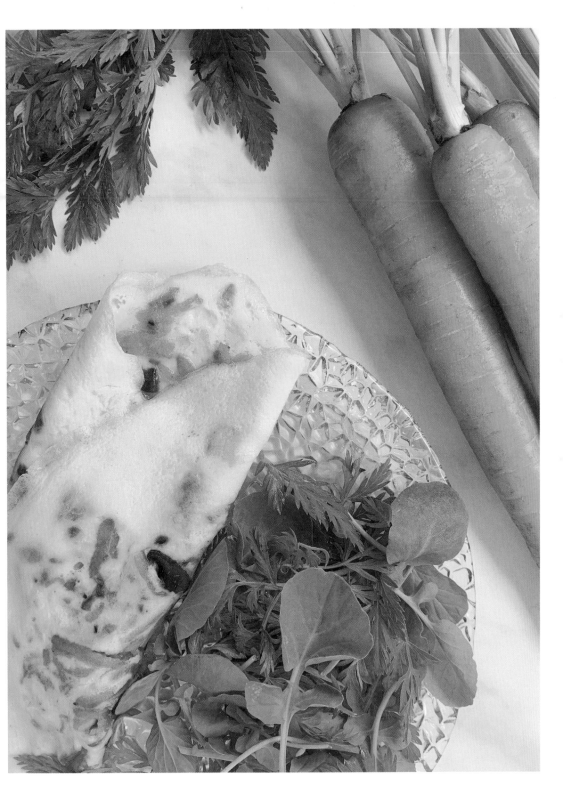

Green Beauty Broth

I adore this recipe for its resourcefulness: the energizing, nutrient-dense base of this broth is essentially made from the scraps of the soup vegetables that you might otherwise toss. It was inspired by a beloved spring soup recipe by vegetarian cooking expert Deborah Madison, and has become a staple breakfast (often paired with a hard-boiled, pastured egg for extra protein) in both warm and cool weather.

MAKES 6 SERVINGS

BROTH BASE

0.5 ounce/15 g dried shiitake mushrooms (about 6)

1 organic celery rib, roughly chopped

Tough ends from 1 bunch asparagus

Dark greens from 2 leeks, roughly chopped

3 garlic cloves

1 bay leaf

½ teaspoon unrefined salt

10 cups/2.4 L water

BROTH

2 tablespoons/30 g grass-fed organic butter or ghee

2 leeks, white and light green parts, chopped

4 garlic cloves, minced

1 bunch asparagus, roughly chopped

2 organic celery ribs, roughly chopped

½ cup packed/30 g fresh parsley leaves and stems, roughly chopped

shiitake mushrooms reserved from broth base, roughly chopped

¾ teaspoon unrefined salt

7 cups broth base

2 large packed handfuls organic arugula

Prepare the broth base: In a medium pot, combine all the broth base ingredients, bring to a boil, lower the heat, and then simmer for 20 minutes. At the 20-minute point, remove the pot from the heat. Remove shiitake mushrooms with a slotted spoon, chop roughly, and set aside. Strain out and discard the other vegetables and bay leaf.

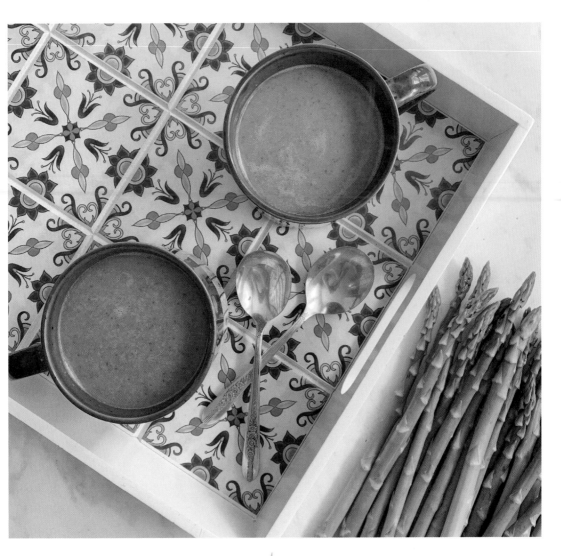

Prepare the broth: In a large pot or Dutch oven, melt the butter over medium heat. Cook the leeks for about 3 minutes, or until they begin to soften. Add the garlic, asparagus, celery, parsley, and chopped mushrooms and cook for 3 minutes more. Add the salt and 7 cups/1.7 L of the broth base, bring to a boil, and simmer until the celery and asparagus soften, about 5 minutes. Remove from the heat and add the arugula. Purée the soup in batches in a high-powered blender. Serve warm or reheat individual servings for a nourishing breakfast.

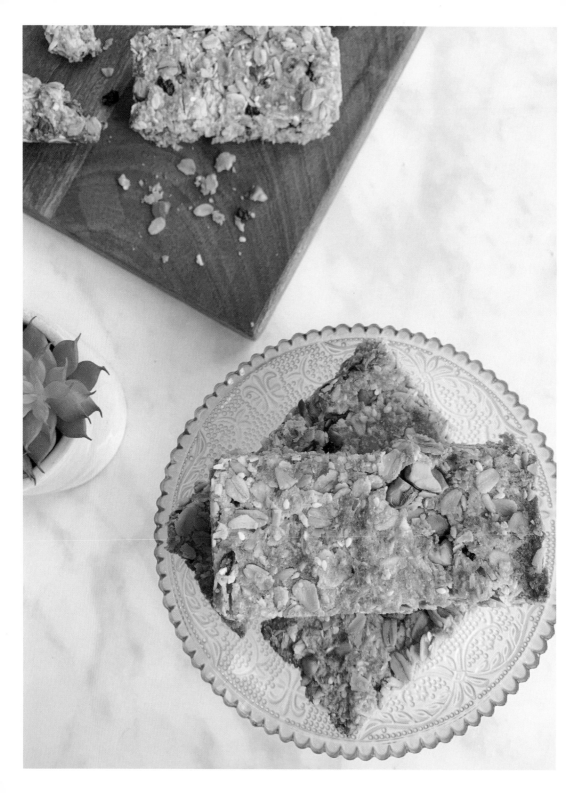

Sesame Glow Bars

Processed and packaged snacks are so convenient, but they rarely leave me with the energy or the fullness that I desire. In their place, I make easily portable snacks, such as these bars that are perfect to grab and go in the morning or any other time of day.

MAKES 8 TO 10 BARS

1 cup packed/180 g pitted dates

1½ cups/150 g gluten-free rolled oats

¾ cup/80 g blanched almond flour

½ cup/50 g unsweetened coconut flakes

2 tablespoons/20 g sesame seeds

2 tablespoons/20 g shelled pistachios, roughly chopped

1 tablespoon/10 g cacao nibs

Scant ¼ teaspoon unrefined salt

½ cup/120 g sesame tahini

⅓ cup/80 g coconut oil, at room temperature

1 teaspoon pure vanilla extract

Preheat the oven to 350°F/180°C. If the dates are not soft and sticky, soak them in hot water for 5 minutes, then drain well.

In a large bowl, mix together the oats, almond flour, coconut flakes, sesame seeds, pistachios, cacao nibs, and salt. In a high-powered blender or food processor, combine half of the dates with the tahini, coconut oil, and vanilla and blend until the mixture begins to form a paste. Add the rest of the dates, a little at a time, blending until smooth. (The paste may separate a little; this is fine.) Add the date paste to the dry ingredients and use a spoon or clean hands to incorporate until the mixture comes together. Press firmly into an 8-inch/20 cm square baking pan. Bake for 20 minutes or until golden brown. Remove from the oven, let cool in the pan, and then cut into bars.

Spring Garden Galette

This savory breakfast is perfect for the freshest vegetables you have on hand. In this version, peppery radishes are cooked until tender and sweet. And don't worry about a cracked or broken crust; you can always patch it up, plus your handmade dish is certain to be filled with love.

SERVES 4

1 cup/130 g buckwheat flour

1 cup/110 g blanched almond flour

1 teaspoon dried thyme

¼ teaspoon unrefined salt

4 tablespoons/60 g plus 1 teaspoon unsalted grass-fed organic butter, divided

5 tablespoons/80 ml water

1 medium-size leek, white and tender green part sliced

2 cups/240 g thinly sliced zucchini

⅔ cup/70 g thinly sliced radishes

Unrefined salt

Freshly ground black pepper

1 tablespoon capers

Organic goat cheese or feta (optional)

Preheat the oven to 350°F/180°C.

In a bowl, stir together the buckwheat flour, almond flour, thyme, and salt. Melt the 4 tablespoons/60 g of butter and add to the flour mixture, stirring to incorporate. Add the water, 1 tablespoon at a time, until the dough sticks together. Form the dough into a ball and roll out to a rough circle of ¼-inch/6 mm thickness in between 2 sheets of parchment paper. Remove the top sheet of parchment, slide the bottom sheet of parchment and crust onto a baking sheet, and set aside.

In a skillet, melt the remaining teaspoon of butter over medium heat and cook the sliced leeks for 1 minute. Add the zucchini and radishes, season with salt and pepper, and cook for about 4 minutes more, or until the vegetables begin to soften. Stir in the capers, then transfer the

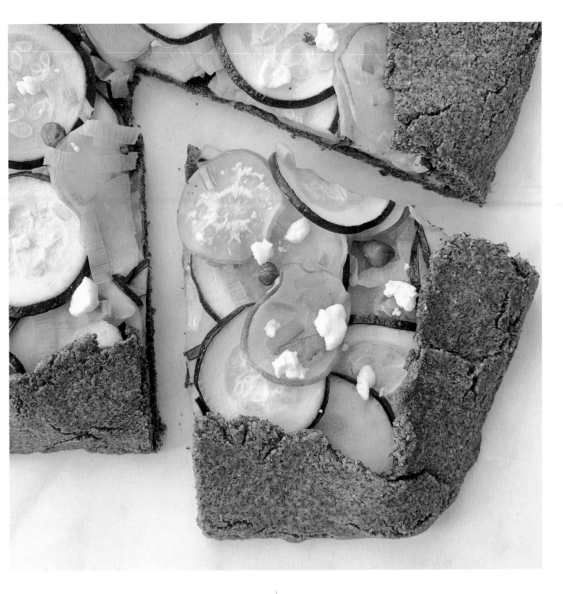

vegetable mixture to the center of the rolled-out dough, piling it high enough to leaving about a 2-inch/5 cm margin of empty dough around the outside. Use your hands to gently fold the bare dough edges, one side at a time, to slightly cover the filling, patching as needed if any breaks occur. Bake for 20 minutes.

Serve warm, topped with a sprinkle of goat cheese or feta, if desired.

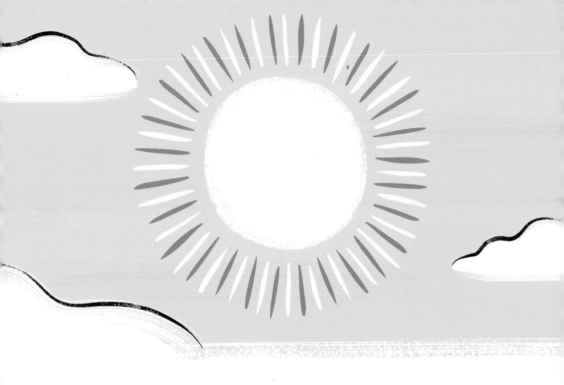

chapter three

Daylight

The sun is high

and the world is abuzz.

Daylight is action time, and so much of your personal energy comes from what you busy yourself with during these midday hours. Building on intensifying sunrise energy, the daylight portion of the day is typically fast-paced, active, dominant, and productive—reflecting the most yang qualities of the 24-hour cycle. Even nature's yang characteristics—bright, sunny, hot—are most likely to surround you during this bustling part of the day.

For your own energetic balance, remember to create moments of calm. When I'm working in my home office, I hear the delicate notes of bells chime through my backyard precisely at noon. The bells, wafting through the air from a church about a mile away, play songs I remember singing as a child. Their soothing effect on my energy is instantaneous. I pause, breathe a little deeper, hum along. This is a perfect cue for me to be present and appreciate the moment where the sun is at its highest point, recharging myself as needed. Try to use the position of the sun or another cue as an energetic reflection point in your own day. The peak of the noon sun is a natural reminder that we're at the most active point in our day, buzzing with energetic potential.

Daylight likely presents the day's biggest opportunity to share your gifts, express your authentic self, and leave the world brighter in your wake. Look around your daylight routine and appreciate the ripple effect of your personal energy on your world. If you could keep an inventory of the people you interact with via touch, words, eye contact, or your expansive personal energy field, that number would be staggering. But even if you interact with only one person a day, your energy is influential. You are a living energetic miracle—a catalyst for *so much power and change* every day, beginning with the people closest to you. There's no doubt that the light you're igniting as you work through each chapter of this book has far-reaching effects. We all have unique ways of sharing our talents and our personal energy, so the only wrong path for this part of your day is one that limits your ability to express your authentic self. The bright energy you created in your morning routine should extend, and amplify, during this part of your day. If something is blocking that, take notice. A valuable daylight energy skill you'll build in this chapter is setting boundaries to protect and preserve your personal energy, while making space for creative flow, uplifting relationships, and continued connection to the wisdom of your body.

DAYLIGHT ENERGY THEMES

creating · building · developing · flowing · experiencing · communicating · connecting · manifesting · interacting

REFLECT ON YOUR DAYLIGHT ENERGY

What are my breaths and stress levels like during the day?

Can I get "in the flow" during my daylight hours?

What are my daily surroundings like?

How long do I sit during the day?

How do I interact with colleagues or clients?

Do I have time to take breaks, and, if so, what do I do with that time?

Do I have a window, or another way to connect my senses to nature?

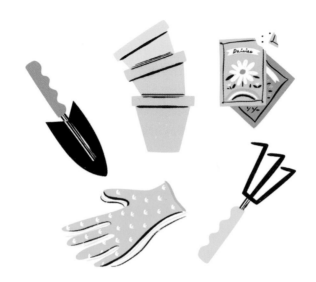

Nature's Energy: Earth and Plants

Amid the busyness of your day, nature's daytime energy elements of earth and plants are the chill pills you've been seeking. If you felt happier, calmer, and more refreshed the last time you hung around in a green space, you weren't imagining things; both the Earth and its plants are deeply grounding to our bodies and soothing to our often overstimulated minds. When something possesses grounding qualities, it conveys feelings of calm, stability, and strength—not unlike the ground itself. The term *grounding* (or *earthing*) also refers to the practice of connecting your body, often the bare soles of your feet, to the Earth to receive a spectrum of impressive energetic benefits.

You probably already know that colorful, fresh, antioxidant-rich foods slow aging free-radical damage in your body. But did you know that grounding has the potential to produce a similar effect, due to the Earth's limitless natural supply of electrons that also neutralize free-radicals? When your skin is electrically connected to (*grounded* by) the electron-rich Earth, study shows you can experience reduced stress and normalized cortisol; an activated parasympathetic nervous system; better circulation (ideally leading to a subsequent boost in skin glow) and wound healing; a 30 percent reduction in pain, stiffness, and soreness; improved sleep; reduced PMS—and lower inflammation and free-radical damage overall. All this, from a low-tech practice that's accessible to all.

To ground your body, kick off your shoes and place your bare feet on dirt, sand, or rocks. Now keep them there (so far, study suggests that 30 minutes is an effective session length), sitting, standing, or even exercising as you wish. Adding water enhances the effect of the electrical connection, so a dewy lawn, wet sand, the ocean floor, or the bottom of a lake or stream are excellent spots to ground your body. Grounding has become one of my go-to ways to balance the frenetic, overstimulated energy I often feel after working on my laptop or phone for an extended period of time (while writing this book, for instance). Sitting or walking with the soles of my feet in grass, dirt, or sand produces a noticeably quieting effect on my nervous system.

If you're a gardener, try grounding yourself with your bare hands in the dirt as you work. Beyond the electron connection, gardening in soil exposes you to beneficial soil-based microbes that strengthen and diversify your microbiome, which helps you stay well and potentially even boosts your mood overall. Surrounded by soil and plants in my garden, I feel such a complete shift toward calm, focused energy. If you enjoy the effects of grounding but you can't be outdoors (say, it's winter where you are), you can purchase modern grounding tools, such as earthing mats, sheets, bands, and shoe inserts, to receive similar energetic effects wherever you are.

If you have access to a forested area of land, you have another free and buzzed-about energetic tool that's increasingly being used as a prescription for healing. Forest bathing, a common practice in Japan and South Korea, involves spending time in a forest setting to quiet and calm the mind and body. Whether you sit, stand, or hike, exposure to the forest environment has a surprising list of energetic benefits. While you're chilling among the trees, you're inhaling phytoncides (essential oils from forest plants, of which there are tens of thousands) that help stimulate serotonin production in the body while increasing natural killer cells, which are key markers of immune function. You're also exposed to a host of microbes that support the health of your own microbiome. I was impressed with the finding of one large-scale study that forest bathing produces a 56 percent increase in natural killer cells on the second consecutive forest bathing session, resulting in a 23 percent increase in immune function that lasted for *a month* even after returning to an urban setting. Other observed benefits include lower cortisol, blood pressure, and heart rate, as well as a 55 percent increase in parasympathetic (relaxing) nervous system function.

Since the body heals best in a relaxed state, simple practices like forest bathing, grounding, and gardening can contribute to big leaps in your physical and energetic health when they become a regular part of your day. Another study found that subjects recovered more quickly from a stressful situation as tree cover in their immediate surroundings increased. The message: seek out some green space (a park, a walking trail, even a picnic bench under a tree) near your workplace or daytime location for daily connection to nature.

Top Daylight Energy Drains

* Working through the day without breaks to reset your energy

* Lacking a balance between solitude and socialization

* Repetitive work that doesn't interest or challenge you

* Skipping lunch and/or regular hydration

* Forgetting to stand up and move around regularly

* Improper breathing and posture

* Sustained levels of high stress

* Lack of opportunities to connect to nature

DAYLIGHT ENERGY INFLUENCERS

Just as the words you speak to another person set off a series of thoughts, reactions, and plans that ripple outward to many others, the energy of others spreads to you, leaving you more vulnerable to outside energy influences during this interactive part of the day. The work you do, people you collaborate with, the environment you spend the day in, and even the other bodies you pass on the street all have the potential to influence your energy. In this section, we'll continue to build your energy awareness to help you avoid being weighed down by dim energy influences across the day. One of my most relied-upon techniques for balancing the barrage of outside energy during the day is to take more frequent moments to turn inward—often through meditation or breath. Ahead, we'll look at the power behind three governing aspects of our daylight energy: work/creativity, relationships/connection, and the energy of our breath, the autonomic function that can become a conscious tool to support energetic well-being.

IN THE FLOW: THE ENERGY OF WORK AND CREATIVITY

So, what do you do all day? You might have a formal, structured job; you might be in school learning and pursuing the career of your dreams; you might have an occupation that requires you to be on call around the clock (hello, parenthood); or some other unique combination of these. To discuss the ways that we're universally affected by the energy of these diverse activities, I'll call them all "work." The work that occupies you all day is a massive energy influencer for four key reasons:

1) **Work often takes up the majority of your waking time (affecting your energy throughout that time and beyond).**

2) **It has the tendency to shape a vital part of your identity.**

3) **It's one big area of your life where you may be able to cultivate positive flow (more on that ahead).**

4) **Your work often connects you to people or places (not always by choice) that become additional energy influencers in your life.**

For most of us, what we do all day is also the means to so many of the other experiences and things we desire from our lives. When it comes to the energy of life, work looms large.

In addition to helping others, work has been my primary path toward two very different experiences: creativity and accomplishment. While both ignite my light, they produce two distinct end results. The creative process is my go-to route to reach a blissful mental state of focused attention called flow. Flow is an incredible promotor of learning, satisfaction, joy, and further creativity—and I want to teach you to use it daily! In moments of flow you can think of your inner light shining as brightly as a lighthouse beacon. And activating this kind of creativity doesn't just feel good in the moment; even brief moments of creative activity have been shown to produce lasting positive emotions, such as excitement and enthusiasm, in addition to feelings of greater purpose and social connection. And the more you express yourself creatively, the more you build your energy.

My type A personality also gets an energetic boost from checking boxes and seeing a task to its successful completion. Achievement is a big part of the energy boost I get from my work—yet it's not that way for everyone. For a little more insight on the way your work affects your energy, make a list of the energetic boosts that you derive from your workday experience. They could include connections, accomplishments, creative outlets, travel and social opportunities, or financial freedom. Get clear on what it is that lights you up in the workspace, and then decide how you can develop more of those aspects of work in your day. It's so essential to recognize that work can actually *work for you*, energetically, if you let it.

Find Your Flow

Before I became a beauty writer, I worked in fashion editorial at a few different magazines. Even as an entry-level intern or assistant, I remember waking up each morning absolutely giddy with excitement to go to work in the fashion closet for the day. The hours (they were long, nonstop, and I was on my feet in heels virtually all day) absolutely flew by. My inner light was blazing because I had found work that tapped both creative and analytical parts of my brain, and also because I was surrounded with so much bright energy, from a group of powerful women who were passionate, creative, and supportive. I felt that energy again when I started my career as an author. Typing page after page in my home office has a vastly different feel from the chaotic floor of a fashion magazine, but the energetic effect is similar for me, with energy being influenced by the environment I've created in my workspace, and the flow state that my brain enters when I'm writing and creating.

Whatever you find yourself doing during the daylight hours, look for opportunities to get in the flow. Flow, or flow state, is the blissed-out, lost-track-of-time feeling that you get when you lose yourself fully in an activity. It's akin to finding your brain's sweet spot in whatever you do. Why does flow feel so amazing? For one, it's a state of balance between sympathetic and parasympathetic nervous system activity. Your senses are heightened, yet your body is relaxed. Picture an ideal yin and yang harmony. During flow, your brain is flooded with a mix of performance and pleasure-enhancing neurotransmitters such as dopamine, norepinephrine, and serotonin that combine relaxation with the ability to focus intently. Occasionally during a flow state, you'll also experience fleeting moments that cause a spiritual feeling—a "wow" effect that is nothing short of blissful.

The entry point to flow has been described as the state in between anxiety (when you're in over your head) and boredom (when a task is way too easy); it's the ideal middle ground. Benefits include a massive boost in creativity (estimated to be 500 percent to 700 percent!), the ability to put aside fears that may otherwise interrupt your action, faster learning, and improved memory. In general, flow is one big "aah" for your brain, which is otherwise engaged in constant, rapid-fire tasks. Flow has become more and more elusive for many of us, given that we are constantly multitasking or plagued by distraction; our collective ability to concentrate has plummeted. But flow state can counter that. **Flow is the energy-shifting Zen moment our busy brains need, one that can actually contribute to a more meaningful existence.**

Which type of work is the best for flow state? Flow can be highly personal, so take note of which activities most often allow you to tune out the world and get completely lost in your work. A few signs that you've been in flow: time seems to speed up or slow down, and you realize that you've had complete concentration (no in-your-head ruminating) on your task. Happily, we don't need a classically creative pursuit, like painting or writing, to get us to a flow state. You can enter flow while changing the oil in a car, folding clothes, or organizing your cabinets. To get started, try a few of these activities that commonly encourage flow:

Drawing or design work	*Sewing or needlepoint*	*Reading*
Dancing	*Viewing art*	*Cooking*
Assembling a puzzle	*Playing an instrument*	*Journaling*

If you know the feeling of counting the minutes until the end of the workday or school day—when it feels like each loop of the second hand is impossibly slow—then you'll appreciate what flow state has to offer. You know how it feels to lose track of time in the midst of an activity, only to realize that an hour or more has passed while you were immersed in a state of focus? The difference between the sluggish ticking of the second hand and the swift, easy passage of an hour can be related to the activity you're doing at the time, as well as flow state.

To make it more likely that you'll enter a flow state in your workday, and stay there as long as you can, try these tips:

* Seek out an activity that grabs your attention and match its level of challenge with your level of skill. As your skills increase with practice, challenge yourself more.

* Minimize distractions as much as possible. If you're working on a computer, turn off e-mail and other notifications. Silence your phone or turn it to airplane mode.

* Put an IN THE FLOW, DO NOT DISTURB sign on your office door. If you tend to get up and move around or get distracted a lot, set a timer for a longer period of time that you want to stay focused.

* If you like music while you work, choose something pleasurable but not distracting.

* Set a reasonable goal and try to exceed it.

* Use aromatherapy, like mint or citrus, which simulates mental focus (see box on page 110).

* Give yourself space. Blocking out time on your calendar for open-ended creative experimentation can help you enter a flow state as you brainstorm and create.

* Relaxed breathing may be a foundation of the flow state; deepen your breathing and read more about breath's influence on energy ahead.

FOCUS ON SCENT

Diffuse these natural scents in your office for optimal energy and focus:

MINT: *supports attention*

CITRUS: *awakens the senses*

CINNAMON: *soothes while increasing alertness*

ROSEMARY: *helps reduce exhaustion and fatigue*

SANDALWOOD: *encourages mental clarity*

Even if you become an expert at focused concentration or flow state, you'll likely find that you begin to lose steam at moments during your day. Take this as a signal to break and replenish your energy, which often needs resetting based on the ultradian rhythm of your own body. Ultradian rhythms are cycles of high and low energy and focus that usually happen in the body every 90 to 120 minutes. Instead of fighting through a low point in your ultradian cycle (and reaching for coffee or sugar to get you through), take a break that allows you to move around, detach completely from what you were working on, and rest your mind. Try a breathing exercise, a guided meditation, a walk, a chat with a friend. Walks are among my favorite breaks because they answer the body's need for movement and support the mental relaxation that lets new thoughts arise. I've come up with my best coaching ideas and some of my favorite book passages while walking. Bring your phone or a journal along so you can record your ideas.

Have you heard the saying that happiness breeds success?
Cultivating satisfaction, joy, and bright energy around your work is so often the first step toward achieving major workplace goals. Energy matters in the workplace—and *every* place.

Workplace Energy Drains

Like all of the other energy influencers in this book, your work and creative outlets can be energy-enhancing friends, or energy-draining foes. Their roles can change at any time, so it's your own ability to navigate energetic highs and lows that becomes essential. In contrast to the energy-building, beacon-of-light-shining flow state is energy depletion. And unfortunately, that's a feeling that so many of us associate with work. After a day's work, it's totally natural to feel spent; to reach a limit where you cannot output anything additional, especially if your job involves physical work. But you don't need to have a physical job to exhaust your body.

Working at a computer in particular can bring on a fog of exhaustion that's a result of long periods of mental processing, electromagnetic fields given off by your computer, and eye fatigue. If you sit at a computer for much of your day, set boundaries that allow you to replenish your energy often. Drink plenty of pure water, move around and refocus your eyes away from a screen regularly, and take periodic breaks to quiet your mind and lower your levels of the stress hormone cortisol.

If you're consistently feeling wholly depleted or exhausted during or after work, some aspect of your work or work environment is draining you unnecessarily. A few scenarios that can be particularly draining for your energy: a difficult co-worker; a task that feels monotonous, stressful, or unstimulating; and a workspace or conditions that are uncomfortable. Any of these sound familiar? With some effort it's likely that you can shift the energy balance. First, set clear energy boundaries in the workplace. Don't think of boundaries as walls that distance you from connection, view them as the tools that help you be healthier, happier, and better understand your needs and the needs of others. When you feel the onset of an energy drain, practice those three R's from Chapter 1: Remove yourself, Release the dim energy, and Reset with one of your instant shifts.

If you have the ability, take steps to change or correct perpetual drains at work (think: bring some music into your workspace, hold more walking meetings to get your body moving, or delegate a task that is dragging down your energy).

While you're at it, build brighter energy into your workplace surroundings. Create a visual inspiration board, incorporate elements of nature into your space, or collect objects that cue you to replenish your energy throughout the workday. Aligning the value of your work output with the importance of the energetic health of your body will only help you perform better and feel more satisfaction in your daylight hours. If you need more of a break from your work, give yourself time to take a mental health day, to not produce anything, to just be, and you'll make space for new ideas. Although the daylight hours are known for being productive, time off helps replenish your energy for tomorrow.

TECH STRESS

While it's still a subject of heated debate, there's evidence to suggest that exposure to the electromagnetic fields given off by computers and smartphones (as well as tons of other appliances and devices around the home and workplace) causes constant, low-grade stress on the body. Although you may or may not be sensitive enough to feel that stress day to day, it can lead to chronically elevated biomarkers, such as inflammation, blood sugar, adrenaline, and cortisol, that deplete your energetic reserves and factor into other more complicated health issues. If your body struggles with outside exposure to electromagnetic fields, you can take steps to reduce your exposure and protect your energy, especially in your own home. The first one: put your phone on airplane mode and shut down your wireless router at night to turn off Wi-Fi!

My biggest workplace energy shift came when:
I started focusing on a single task for an extended period of time, allowing me to concentrate and enter a flow state more often.

Finding Your Purpose at Work

What if the work you do all day is not the work that lights you up? I don't know a single person who hasn't grappled with this question at one time or another. If life's work and the creativity journey were all sunshine and heart-eye emojis, we definitely wouldn't be talking about them here. I think the answer to this universal question is unique to each of us. There will be times when you have bright energy flowing through every other area of your life, and feeling out of your element during your workday won't be enough to upset your energetic balance. But maybe all at once you're faced with an injury that limits your movement, a stressful relationship, and construction going on in your home. Your energy sources shift. The effects of dim energy at work become harder to shoulder when bright energy is not readily flowing from other areas. Feeling dim energy at work is especially challenging because so many of us spend such a substantial portion of our lives in a working role, and when that role aligns with our identity or higher purpose, it helps us feel lit from within.

Try to view your work situation with fresh eyes and possibility—perhaps your current work is short term; a stepping stone on a path that's leading you somewhere brighter. Perhaps it enables you to do or be what you truly love during the other times of your day, especially if you have another creative outlet that brings you joy. And perhaps you derive satisfaction from your work, without needing to feel passionate purpose. In any of those situations, I firmly believe you can still maintain enough positivity around your work to let it be an energetic plus in your life. And if or when you decide it's time for a change, let your energy be a guide to your next role. Trust that it's never off limits for you to follow energy in a new direction, learn a new skill, reinvent yourself, and find the working role that better fits your higher purpose.

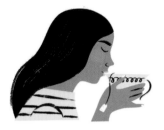

WORK/CREATIVE ENERGY IN PRACTICE: MINDFUL SINGLE-TASKING

The workday, and the world, move quickly and constantly. One deadline begets another; even weekends come with to-do lists. And given ever-updating social media and news feeds, your brain and body bounce around from thought to task to action during every waking hour. One recent study found that people spend 47 percent of their waking hours thinking about something other than what they're currently doing, and that constant mind wandering breeds unhappiness. To counter this frenetic pace, lower your reactivity, and raise the calm, creative energy of your body (while still allowing you to get stuff done); there's no antidote like single-tasking. This is a great example of doing less to achieve more. Pouring your attention into a single focused task turns your brain from a messy jumble to a clear, organized, productive machine. You'll be surprised how efficient your single-tasking brain becomes.

Single-tasking sounds easy, but you might be surprised at its challenges. Remember the last time you tried to clear your mind and meditate? Thoughts and distractions probably came flying at you from all directions. Expect something similar when you single-task. Do your best to shut out distractions to prevent interruption, which *significantly* increases the amount of time it takes to complete a task (it's likely the number one drain on your productivity). And before you take on your next task, give yourself a moment of rest. Truly resting before starting another activity can make you more focused and productive.

10 Activities to Single-Task

Choose just one at a time and focus on being present and enjoying the process, with no distractions:

1) Cook a meal.

2) Fold laundry.

3) Shower, paying attention to each action as you complete it.

4) Keep only one tab open on your Internet browser.

5) Walk with no earbuds, just enjoying the activity and your surroundings.

6) Sit down and write someone a letter from start to finish.

7) Read a book.

8) Sip a cup of tea or a glass of wine and really savor its flavors.

9) Play a board game.

10) Have a conversation with a friend.

⇒ Energy Booster ⇐

The color green enhances visual creativity, and the creative boost your brain gets from green actually takes effect in only a few seconds. Keep a green plant or another green object at your desk for inspiration. Better yet, get outside and into green space when you need a creative wakeup; nature not only boosts and refreshes brain function, time in nature has been shown to help break through creative blocks.

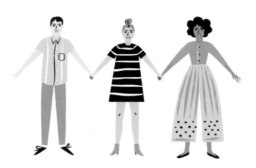

COME TOGETHER:
THE ENERGY OF RELATIONSHIPS
AND CONNECTION

When you reflect on the energy influencers that color happiness, health, and your overall life experience, you begin to realize that you, yourself, are an energy influencer in the lives of so many people. You—as you are right here, right now—are an energy conduit. You convey energy not only in words and actions but in your presence, facial expressions, posture, gestures, and touch. Remember your vibrational energy field, the one that extends several feet from your body? That field is constantly interacting and exchanging energy with those around you (this includes animals, as well as people). And through your energetic exchanges, you're influencing someone else's existence—health, mood, joy, even beauty—as they're influencing yours. If we zoom out and look at the world at large, it's clear that **every energy exchange serves as an opportunity to light up someone else and create or continue an energetic ripple effect that holds the potential to grow to a massive scale.** This likely makes the energy of your relationships and connections your single biggest opportunity to create change every day. You have the personal power to ignite your light and then spread it to everything in this life. And you don't have to be a shaman, a meditation expert, or yogi to access this power.

I love Maya Angelou's observation that "People will forget what you said, people will forget what you did, but people will never forget how you made them feel." That feeling is energy. So, how *do* you make others feel? What energetic effect do you leave in your wake? Personal energy is a choice, one that you reaffirm hundreds of times over the course of a single day. You don't need a podium or red carpet to make a profoundly positive shift; start in your workspace, among your friends, in the next interaction you have. In doing so, as you'll read ahead, you'll create a ripple of energy that impacts others in addition to building beauty, joy, and fulfillment that returns to your own life.

The millions of energetic exchanges made every day don't have a hierarchy of value. The only way to make an energetic exchange more significant is to pass it on, allowing it to proliferate. If we were all to meet that simple goal of spreading brighter energy among our daily essentials, the resulting energetic shift would be staggering. So, why not start today? Spreading bright energy doesn't have to be as involved as gifting a bouquet of flowers or treating a friend to lunch; you spread light simply by embodying it yourself (another reason that your mindset alone holds so much power and influence). Scientific study has shown that happiness, for example, spreads readily through social networks, families, and friends in close proximity. In fact, your happiness alone makes it 34 percent more likely that your next-door neighbor will be happy. Imagine the brightening effect that has on the happiness of your street, your community, and the world!

Personal energy spreads in much the same way; it's contagious and it causes a vibrational shift in those around you. Remember, the vibrations of objects in close proximity often sync up. They literally begin to vibrate together. Any action that you take to make someone else's day brighter becomes the ultimate energy boost, shifting your own energy in turn. Today, seek out more opportunities to purposefully bring light to others, and feel an even greater shift take place within you as a result. Such an act is not about people-pleasing, it's about creating a better experience for everyone, since its light flows to both sides. The next time you feel overwhelmed and powerless to fix a negative social or political situation, start a ripple effect by *being* the light. Immerse yourself in the potential of your relationships rather than the feeling of overwhelm.

CHANGE THE ENERGY OF A ROOM

The next time you need to stand in front of a group for a speech, lecture, performance, or even just to ask a question, think about the opportunity that you have to shift the energy of the entire room with your own. The fastest way to put a whole room at ease and in a more positive headspace is with a visual: your facial expression. Thanks to the brain's mirroring effect, which helps us empathize, we tend to reflect and experience the same emotions displayed in the facial expressions of others. The downside is that in a negative interaction we can walk away with unwanted energy that becomes our own. But a relaxed smile spreads the energy of ease and actually makes you calmer, as a signal to your brain that releases happiness neurotransmitters. Its effect can completely change the experience of your message, and help your audience walk away feeling brighter!

Energy Attracts

Creating positive change in our world is reason enough for most of us to strive to light ourselves up. But there is another appealing reason that consciously choosing to embody bright energy is worth your effort: energy is a major attractive force. Bright energetic qualities, such as kindness, thoughtfulness, compassion, humbleness, patience, courage, and love, are not only uplifting—they're magnetic. Here's another place where our cultural pursuit of peak beauty overlaps with this conversation about energy: bright energy is a beauty secret for the ages. I've questioned and explored this for over a decade as a beauty editor—what is it that makes someone magnetic, attractive, and desirable, independent of physical appearance? It's energy. Yes, I'm saying that the most beautiful thing about you may be more of a feeling than a visible feature.

Beauty, magnetism, and attraction involve far more than the physical traits that so many of us relentlessly pursue. Beauty is inherently physical *and* energetic. You may be able to judge physical beauty in a social media post or magazine ad, but in person you'll find a much broader assessment of beauty—perhaps one that repels or attracts you, depending on energy. So, what energy is the most attractive to you? I find energy that's fresh, vibrant, and youthful (in spirit, though not predicated on age) lights up a room and leaves a lasting impression.

I JUST DON'T FEEL POSITIVE

At times, our energy is just not what we want it to be. We feel stuck, sad, sick, frustrated, or just plain bored with the status quo. If that's you today, feel that energy and let it move you toward a change. And when you're ready, release that feeling to make room for what's new and next in your life. During years of chronic illness, I often found myself needing to express my dim energy (usually in the form of worries or fears) out loud, but after doing so I was almost instantly able to release it. When speaking my fears didn't seem helpful to myself or others, I learned to express them in prayer, which enabled me to release them as well. For more ways to release, see page 206.

If dim energetic states become a pattern in your life, it helps to periodically step back and reflect honestly on the energy that you're putting out into the world. Have a candid talk with a close friend or two about the energy you convey and how it makes them feel. If it's not the energy that you desire at this moment in your life, you're reading the right book. As you pass through your day, look for the root source or sources of dim energy, whether internal or external, that affect you. Although you won't be able to change every circumstance, you *can* shift your mindset and your relationship with that source.

Surround Yourself with the Energy You Want

As humans, we're built to connect. But we forget, or simply aren't conscious, that human connection is more than a by-product of living on a planet with 7 billion other people—it's a biological need that affects our lives in the deepest ways. The mere presence of another person has incredible, yet invisible, influence over you, affecting your immune system, your mood, your brain, your cells, and even your genes. When touch, dialogue, or other experiences are exchanged along with energy, the influence grows. Positive social relationships also turn on our parasympathetic nervous system, making them a seriously undervalued tool for aging well, hormone balance, healing, longevity, and stress relief. Thus far, social experiments suggest that gathering with friends just twice a week has notable health benefits, including faster recovery from illness, a stronger immune system, lower anxiety, and even increased generosity. Strong family and friend relationships reduce your risk of dying from illness by 50 percent—largely from reductions in stress, inflammation, and fear that would otherwise suppress the immune system.

Of course, when you're in the midst of a struggle, you don't like where you are in life, or you're not feeling your best, it's easy to retreat from social connections. The answer is often to seek out supportive relationships that surround you with the energy you want to possess. Connecting with others who practice or possess what you're looking to achieve can help you get there. In short, you start to mirror who you spend time with. Scientific study has found that simply watching or reading about someone striving toward a goal makes you more likely to adopt that goal yourself. There's also growing evidence that your energetic power is amplified many times when you sync up your intentions with others. Consider how you can increase your own energetic potential to create positive change by aligning yourself with people who are like-minded. Just the same, keeping the company of people who spread dim energy threatens your own light along with the beauty, health, resilience, and joy in the life you're consciously building. In many cases, the effect of someone else's behavior on your own might be incredibly subtle— something you aren't even conscious of until you shift away.

QUESTIONS TO ASK WHILE ASSESSING ANOTHER PERSON'S ENERGETIC ROLE IN YOUR LIFE:

How do I feel after spending time with this person?

Do I trust this person fully?

Does this person support my energetic heath in the present moment?

Do I have chemistry with, or feel a strong connection to, this person?

Is our relationship balanced in terms of energy exchange?

BEWARE THE ENERGY VAMPIRE

A so-called energy vampire is a human energy drain who continually sucks the bright energy out of others, leaving a state of negativity or dim energy. They might be well intentioned and generally good—and they may even be a close friend or family member—but they don't help you toward your goal of growing the light in your life. And they deliver negativity that can become detrimental to your physical health and beauty. You don't need to (and many times you can't) remove this person from your life, but you can set boundaries on how much they affect your energy.

Fielding Negativity

One of the truths of our experience as humans is that we can never fully understand the life experience of another person. We don't know what it feels like to inhabit their physical body, to receive all of the varied energy influencers that they encounter in their days. Although you can't completely understand or control the energy that others possess, you always have the choice whether

121

or not to change *your* energy. Next time you receive negativity from another person, rather than reacting right away, pause. Breathe. Reserve judgment. Remember that this person is human, just like you. Consider where this person's words or actions might be coming from (a place of defensiveness, anger, fear—even a ripple of dim energy from someone else?). Aim not to take this negativity personally, and remember that it's not your responsibility to change anyone. If needed, respond in a way that allows your own bright energy to shine through. Know that often, listening alone may be the best way to help someone else release dim energy.

Above all, don't perpetuate that dim energetic state. To take care of yourself in that situation, you might even imagine yourself surrounded by protective energy, with your own bright light keeping you from the dark. Being a voice of compassion and kindness for yourself allows you to be that for others, too. Practice the three R's on page 40, and if this negativity dump happens repeatedly, speak up about the way you feel.

My biggest relationship energy shift came when:
I gave myself permission to steer clear of people whose dim energy continually drains my own while healing.

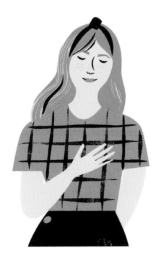

RELATIONSHIPS AND CONNECTION
ENERGY IN PRACTICE: REIKI

Did you know that simply placing a hand over your heart, or anywhere that feels soothing to you, while you take a few deep breaths, releases oxytocin and naturally occurring opiates that lower your own cortisol levels? You can produce the same effect in others as you share your healing energy.

The Japanese healing practice of Reiki (meaning "healing energy") is one of the best demonstrations of the energy that can pass from person to person. Reiki is based on the transference of energy, and it involves hands-on touch or near touch to improve the energy of mind, body, and spirit. Benefits of Reiki found in scientific study include reduction in pain, fatigue, and anxiety; increase in heart rate variability (a measure of stress recovery); and a boost in positive emotions. Recipients of Reiki report deep relaxation and a profound sense of healing. Most recently, scientific study has shown that Reiki significantly surpasses a placebo in its ability to activate the parasympathetic nervous system, supporting mind-body healing.

If you seek out a professional Reiki session, a trained Reiki practitioner will place his or her hands (hands are known to be particularly strong energetic connection points) on or slightly above you to transfer energy that supports your body's own well-being and healing processes. If you're healing from a broken arm, you may find that your practitioner focuses his or her hands on the site of your injury. Or you may receive broader, head-to-toe Reiki for a boost in total well-being. I encourage you to try professional Reiki (there are over 4 million practitioners in the world—perhaps even someone you already know), especially if you feel the need for more positive personal connections in your life.

But even before you experience Reiki, you can experiment with energy transference that supports healing and well-being right now, wherever you are. Try this alone, or with a friend. Start with a relaxed breath and a mindset that supports healing, well-being, and calm. To feel the power and energy in your hands, rub them together for a minute. Hold your hands a few inches apart, palms facing each other, and feel any energy that passes between them. Place your hands on an area of your body, or your friend's body, that needs healing. If you're just experimenting with energy without a healing purpose, try the heart, the upper chest (sternum area), or the sides of the head as focus points. As you hold your hands there, breathe deeply and slowly. Visualize warm golden light passing through your body, down your arms, into your hands, and into his or her body, and repeat an affirmation that focuses your mind on bright energy, like "May you feel peace, comfort, and abundant health." If you're trying this on yourself, imagine that the energy is flowing into you through the crown of your head, flowing to your hands, and then into the spot where your hands are resting. After a few minutes (aim for 15 for more pronounced benefits), end your session. Incredibly, research suggests that the transfer of electromagnetic waves that occurs through this simple laying on of hands technique positively benefits immune cells.

Many feel strongly that you can use this same technique to exchange energy without being face-to-face. Recall that quantum theory says that connections can exist even if two objects are separated by immense distance. You are connected to others, to the earth, to nature, to all of the wonders and mysteries of the universe, giving you massive power to create change, even among people you aren't physically close to. If you indeed have connections to everything and everyone, why not experiment with spreading healing and love to someone far away from you who needs it today? Rather than using your hands directly, visualize that healing light transmitting from your body, across the miles to the person in need. While transmitting healing energy may sound improbable, distance-healing has already been shown to be effective in randomized controlled trials in humans, animals, plants, bacteria, yeast, and even DNA.

⪢ Energy Booster ⪡

Although social media often makes us feel hyperconnected, it also displaces opportunities for the face-to-face interactions that are so integral to our well-being. When social media connections overtake in-person ones, we run the risk of increasing our loneliness—an emotional and energetic state that has real, negative physical effects on the body. I've found so many upsides to social media, but they don't replace the energy I receive from time spent with friends or family. It's through those in-person connections that we exchange energy, sync our vibrations, and spread energetic change. As you explore the power of relationships and connection, remember your energetic needs and seek out the valuable personal connections that fulfill you most.

NITIKA'S DAYLIGHT

NAME: Nitika Chopra

WHAT TO KNOW ABOUT ME:
I create content that teaches people how to love themselves, with a focus on the chronic illness community. I love to sing in the Resistance Revival Chorus, and I have psoriasis and psoriatic arthritis.

THE DAYLIGHT HOURS OF MY DAY ARE USUALLY:
Energized.

MY ESSENTIALS FOR THE BEST DAYLIGHT ENERGY:
Surrounding myself with people who are as passionate about their lives as I am; plus a solid 7 hours of sleep, a great oat milk latte, and jewelry that shows my sparkle.

FAVORITE WAY TO FUEL MY BODY DURING DAYLIGHT HOURS:
I eat an autoimmune Paleo diet that keeps me in optimal health; I love munching on macadamia nuts and seaweed snacks during the day.

DAYLIGHT ENERGY INFLUENCERS AFFECT MY PERSONAL ENERGY MOST IN THE AREA OF:
Relationships. I feel like my connection to a higher power is the thing that anchors me and fuels me most. And I find the reflection of God, a higher power, and all that is good and possible in the world is most apparent to me when I'm connecting with like-minded people. Healthy relationships are my nonnegotiable; they are my life source energy.

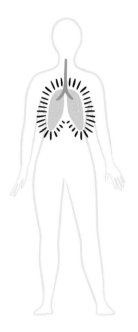

YOUR ANCHOR FOR CALM: THE ENERGY OF BREATH

If your brain is the composer, and your heart the metronome, then your breath is surely the conductor of your body's energetic orchestra. You take an average of 23,000 breaths every day. Each has its own modest effect on your body, but collectively those thousands of breaths have the potential to completely transform your personal energy. Not only do they keep you alive, but those breaths help you respond to thoughts, situations, and surroundings. **Changing your breathing pattern is one of the fastest ways to shift your consciousness.** With simple, purposeful alterations in your breath, you send direct messages to your body: messages of calm and safety, excitement and fear, focus and alertness. Your breath informs your physical body much like your thoughts. But most of us could stand a little education and even retraining around those 23,000 daily breaths. In this section, you'll learn key ways to shift your breath to influence the state of your body in minutes. Practice them, incorporate them daily, and you'll discover that you hold energetic influence over your body even in highly emotional situations.

Energetically, your breath is life itself. The way you breathe affects your ability to perform mentally and physically, to cleanse waste, and to circulate energy and nutrients. Oxygen is essential for the production of ATP, the molecule that powers our cells. Ideally, we'd all breathe freely, letting breath be intuitive and easy. But so many of us get stuck in a stress-induced state of tight, shallow breathing—one that becomes a sustained negative influence on energy—especially during this part of the day. It's a cyclical problem; a trigger shifts your breath into a depleting pattern that makes you even more vulnerable to dim energetic thoughts and influences. Stopping the cycle requires you to shift your breath pattern back to a state of energetic calm.

Let's grow your breath consciousness by checking on your breathing right now. Sit up straight or lie down and place one hand on your chest, one hand on your abdomen, and breathe in deeply. You should feel your abdomen, the lower part of your torso, move and expand, as well as some subtle movement in your rib cage. If your upper chest is rising or you feel yourself straining to take enough air into your chest, you're sending your body an energetic message of tension and stress. Chest breathing tells your body that it needs to stay alert against threats, and contributes to pain and tension in your neck as it activates upper body muscles. Diaphragmatic breathing, through your lower belly beneath your navel, is a signal of ease and safety that enhances your ability to learn and concentrate. Continue paying attention to your breath for several breath cycles and see whether you can shift to, or maintain, a lower belly breath. Check in with your breath throughout the day and pay attention to triggers that take your breath out of its relaxed pattern. One study showed that simply typing on a keyboard caused participants to chest breathe, increase their rate of breathing, and brace their upper body.

Breathe Calm

The simple act of placing a hand on your abdomen reminds you to breathe from your diaphragm rather than your chest; that may be all you need to reset your breathing in times of stress. But if you have difficulty finding calm, changing the pattern of your breath can help transfer you from fight-or-flight mode into a relaxed, parasympathetic state where recovery and peak energy flow happens. Begin the shift by pausing for one second after you exhale, and then gradually extend the length of each subsequent exhale as long as you feel comfortable. You can do this by counting your breaths in and out (say, 4 counts in and 5 counts out), or by adding a little extra puff of exhale in the pause before you inhale again. As you do so, increase your awareness of your surroundings. Reassure your body that you are safe, right where you are.

When your exhale is longer than your inhale, you stimulate the vagus nerve, the body's longest nerve with multiple branches that travel from your brain down your neck, torso, and through your intestines, linking directly to your heart along the way. Vagus nerve stimulation releases acetylcholine to contract muscles and subsequently calm your nervous system and heart rate. To apply your visualization skills here, picture your vagus nerve wandering down through your abdomen, releasing acetylcholine that is calming you with every exhale. Over time, stimulating the vagus nerve lowers the stress hormone cortisol and reduces inflammation (thereby slowing signs of aging), improves digestion, and even encourages neuroplasticity, allowing you to more readily change your brain patterns.

OTHER WAYS TO ACTIVATE THE VAGUS NERVE

The health of your vagus nerve is not only a key marker of your own energetic health, it actually influences the health and vagal tone of other people you come into contact with. The good news is, you can stimulate your vagus nerve and interrupt your own stress response with more than just long exhales. Add these diverse vagus nerve-activating techniques to your routine for a reduction in inflammation, better digestion, and greater stress resilience, among other benefits. Practice them daily to help yourself default to calm, bright energy over time:

Yoga	*Singing*	*Exercise*	*Gum-chewing*
Meditation	*Laughter*	*Massage*	*Acupuncture*
Humming	*Prayer*	*Fasting*	*Cold Showers*

Breathe Naturally

Next time you want to take in a deeper breath, start by exhaling fully. Increasing your oxygen intake and taking deeper breaths—a goal for so many of us—starts with longer, more complete exhales rather than bigger breaths in. Your breath should naturally have an exhale that's slightly longer than your inhale. If you find yourself straining to take bigger breaths in, you could actually be hyperventilating—a breathing pattern that can be incredibly subtle (you may never suspect that you're doing it) and widespread. When we hyperventilate, even slightly, we produce less carbon dioxide, which is essential to a body in homeostasis. Too little carbon dioxide leads to overactivation of the nervous system, muscle tension, and constriction of blood flow to tissues that can result in headaches, poor concentration, even cold hands and feet, impeding energy flow. If you periodically need to take a big inhale to "catch up" on your breath, this is one sign of slight hyperventilation. Focus on a longer exhale instead, and feel your body relax.

A popular breath pattern that exaggerates the pattern of a shorter inhale and longer exhale to calm the body quickly is the 4-7-8 breath. Remember these numbers and you'll always be able to practice this breath in times of stress or discomfort. Begin by exhaling all of your air. Inhale slowly through your nose for 4 counts, hold that breath in for 7 counts (helping to deeply oxygenate your body), then slowly release your breath through your nose or mouth for 8 counts. Pause and repeat this cycle 3 or 4 times to produce a discernable shift in your energy and fight-or-flight response. This is a perfect breath pattern to practice if you notice daytime stress building in the form of tense muscles, mental distraction, and shallow breaths. It's a breath I use to dispel nervous tension before public speaking or teaching, and I also frequently lead my audiences in this breath because it's such an empowering tool for lowering stress and positively impacting energy, hormone balance, and overall radiance.

It's also beneficial to your energy to get comfortable nose-breathing, and to make sure your nose is your default channel of breath. Taking in air through your nose rather than your mouth when you're at rest (or even during exercise, as some athletes train to do) is calming to the body and helps maintain balance in your autonomic nervous system. This type of breath oxygenates your cells much more fully and completely than a chest breath. That extra oxygen, and subsequent increase in carbon dioxide, supports an incredible cascade of processes that allow you to function at and feel your best.

Nose-breathing has also been linked to increased activity in the parasympathetic nervous system that helps your body digest, repair, and increase detoxifying lymph flow, whereas mouth-breathing has been linked to increased fight-or-flight response, which slows lymph and raises the stress hormone cortisol. Next time you notice yourself mouth-breathing, take a moment to assess your body and see whether you can figure out why. Are you panicky? Is your stress level too high? Is your nose simply stuffed? Switch back to nose-breathing, take a moment to relax your body, and feel your energy shift.

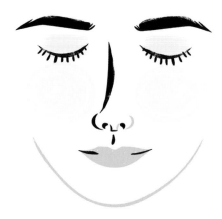

> **My biggest breathing energy shift came when:**
> I started taking breaks to sit outside and slow my breathing
> several times a day.

BREATH ENERGY IN PRACTICE:
NADI SHODHANA

Heightening both relaxation and alertness, nadi shodhana, or alternate nostril breath, is the antidote to the demanding combination of a stressful work environment *and* a workload requiring mental focus that so many of us juggle each day. This breath exercise helps you chill out and snap your brain into concentration mode all at once! Workday benefits of nadi shodhana include a boost in attention and fine motor coordination, coupled with a drop in blood pressure. To practice it, you'll breathe in through one nostril and out through the other, always closing off the opposite nostril that's not taking in or releasing air. Many people use the thumb to gently close off one nostril and the ring finger of the same hand to close off the other nostril during the practice. You can use those fingers, or any that feel comfortable to you.

Start by making sure your nose is clear (skip this practice on days when you have a stuffy nose). Exhale fully, and close off your right nostril with your right thumb.

Breathe in through your left nostril, holding in your breath while you remove your thumb and close off the left nostril with your right ring finger.

Now that your right nostril is open, exhale slowly through it, then inhale slowly through it.

Remove your ring ringer from the left nostril, close off your right nostril with your thumb, and breathe out through your left nostril.

Remember that each time you inhale is a cue for you to switch fingers and nostrils, exhaling your breath out of the opposite side.

With repetition and practice, this breath pattern becomes rhythmic, almost hypnotic in its ability to focus your attention. Aim for 3 minutes of nadi shodhana, and work your way up to 10. You should feel balanced, grounded, and less reactive when you finish. And the benefits extend beyond your energetic state to support of hormone balance and mental output, as this breath is thought to balance the two hemispheres of your brain.

⇒ Energy Booster ⇐

If you sit at a desk most of the day, it's easy to develop poor posture: shoulders that slump, a neck jutting forward, a tight upper back. Poor posture worsens breathing (reducing lung capacity by as much as 30 percent), and poor breathing habits actually worsen posture as well. The good news is that mindfully changing one will help improve the other. Whenever you check in with your breath, take a moment to sit up, straighten your back, and pull your shoulders down and back. Keep your belly relaxed while you breathe in (this helps you take a full breath from your diaphragm). Feel your body strong and relaxed.

SLEEPY, OR TENSE?

If you find yourself yawning or sighing throughout the day, this may be your body's way of dissipating accumulated muscle tension. Let yourself sigh, or exhale slowly as you produce a humming sound, for an instant dose of peaceful energy (read more about the energy of humming on page 175). You'll soon realize that chanting "om" is an energetic tool you can use outside of yoga class as well.

More Ways to Feel the Energy of Daylight

❋ Connect with someone and see where it leads! Have lunch or tea with a coworker or friend, new or old.

❋ Bring work outside. Which activities can you do while staying grounded with the Earth?

❋ Pause all of your activity for a moment and be completely present and still. Appreciate your energetic contribution to this day so you can maximize it.

❋ Note the position of the sun. Is it rising, sinking, or at its pinnacle? Note how that influences your energy in the moment.

❋ Create a connection with a stranger by practicing a random act of kindness. How does it shift your own energy?

RECIPES TO NOURISH YOUR DAYLIGHT ENERGY

Daylight's ideal food sustains a busy, creative period in your schedule with nutrient-dense ingredients, on-the-go fuel, and extra brain support. The act of nourishment often provides opportunities for self-care or connection with others, an important midday energy influencer. You might use your daylight mealtime as an opportunity to fortify yourself with personal energetic connections as well as food. I often seek out daylight nourishment that inspires my own creative expression by exciting my senses with color, flavor, texture, and scent. I also add adaptogens, herbs, and other natural ingredients that help balance the stress response and enable the body to be more resilient during the daylight hours, while protecting overall health and beauty, supporting mental focus, or aiding the healing process. Here you'll find some of my favorite recipes that support daylight energy, from midday meals to productivity-fueling afternoon snacks to keep tucked into your bag or your desk.

Ideal food for daylight energy:
slow-burning fuel that will power your body through a long stretch of activity, like beans and lentils, raw nuts and seeds, protein-rich chickpeas, or wild salmon; mildly stimulating teas or chocolates that encourage energy and focus; ample liquids for hydration

Gingersnap Cashews

Sweet, spicy, and salty, with the buttery flavor of roasted cashews—this addictive and anti-inflammatory snack will jumpstart your daylight hours. I grab a handful as I'm running out the door or keep a bowl at my desk for workday fuel.

MAKES 2 CUPS CASHEWS

2 teaspoons coconut oil, melted

3 tablespoons pure maple syrup

2 teaspoons ground turmeric

2 ¼ teaspoons ground ginger

⅛ teaspoon unrefined salt

2 cups/300 g raw cashews

Preheat the oven to 350°F/180°C. Line a baking sheet with parchment paper. In a bowl, stir together the coconut oil, maple syrup, turmeric, ginger, and salt. Add the nuts and toss to coat. Transfer the nuts to the prepared pan and spread them out evenly. Roast for 12–15 minutes, watching closely to prevent burning, and stirring halfway. Remove from the oven and immediately transfer the nuts off the pan (I like to lift the entire sheet of parchment up and slide it onto a countertop) to cool. Tip: Store in a glass container to prevent staining.

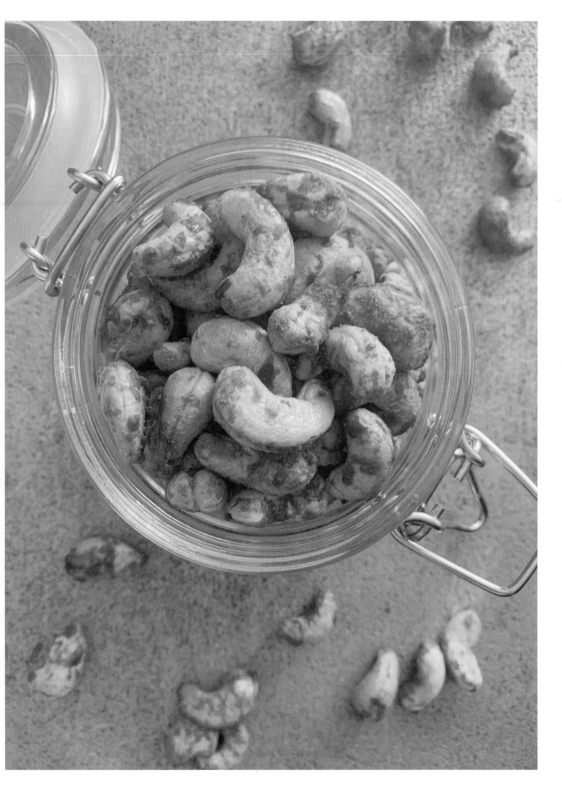

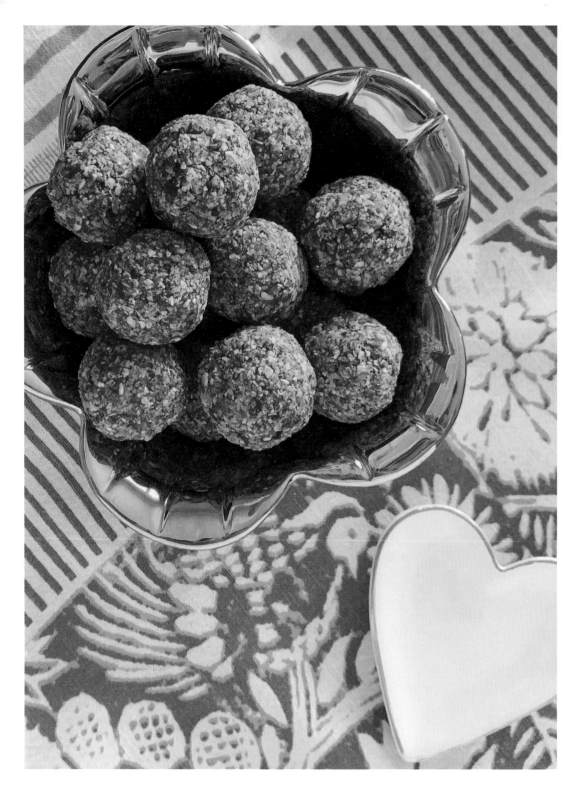

Coconut-Raspberry Love Bites

I aim to spread the energy of love in the food that I make. And these sweet, hand-rolled snacks carry a little love in every bite. I like them as a special treat during the workday, as well as a fun surprise for my son's lunchbox—so he gets a reminder of my love even at school.

MAKES 17 (1-INCH) BALLS

1 cup packed/65 g unsweetened shredded coconut flakes

⅓ cup/40 g organic rolled oats

¼ cup/60 g pitted dates

1 tablespoon coconut oil

½ teaspoon pure vanilla extract

⅛ teaspoon unrefined salt

2 tablespoons/18 g raw almonds

1 tablespoon unsweetened nondairy milk

1 cup/24 g freeze-dried raspberries

In a food processor, combine the coconut, oats, dates, coconut oil, vanilla, and salt and process on high speed for 1-2 minutes, or until a uniform crumbly mixture forms. Add the almonds and milk and pulse until the almonds have broken up. Add the raspberries and pulse again until just incorporated. Roll into 1-inch/2.5 cm balls. Chill and serve. Store in the refrigerator for up to 1 week.

Fueled & Focused Salad with Superfood Sunflower Dressing

The chickpea polenta in this recipe might just become your favorite new protein staple for workday lunches. Atop this salad, its flavors echo bites of nutty, earthy falafel with creamy dressing and fresh veggies. Spicy watercress is one of my favorite greens for its incredible DNA-repairing benefits, and I love how eating it brightens my energy!

SERVES 4

1 cup/150 g chickpea flour

¾ teaspoon unrefined salt

½ teaspoon garlic powder, divided

¼ teaspoon ground cumin

3 cups/750 ml water, plus about 4 teaspoons for dressing

¼ cup/5 g fresh parsley and cilantro leaves, finely minced

¼ cup/80 g sunflower seed butter

¼ cup/62 ml lemon juice

2 tablespoons/20 ml coconut aminos

2 teaspoons whole-grain mustard

1 teaspoon reishi mushroom powder*

4 large handfuls of fresh watercress (about 4 ounces/120 g)

1 cup/150 g tomatoes, chopped

½ cup/60 g sweet bell pepper, seeded and chopped

¼ cup/30 g chopped red onion

2 tablespoons/18 g raw sunflower seeds

In a bowl, stir together the chickpea flour, salt, ¼ teaspoon of the garlic powder, and the cumin. Whisk in 1½ cups/375 ml of the water. In a saucepan, bring the remaining 1½ cups/375 ml of water to a boil. Lower the heat and whisk in the chickpea mixture, stirring frequently until thick and creamy, 3 to 5 minutes. Add the parsley and cilantro and stir to combine. Remove from the heat and spread the polenta mixture in an 8-inch/20 cm square glass pan, then chill for 1 hour in the refrigerator.

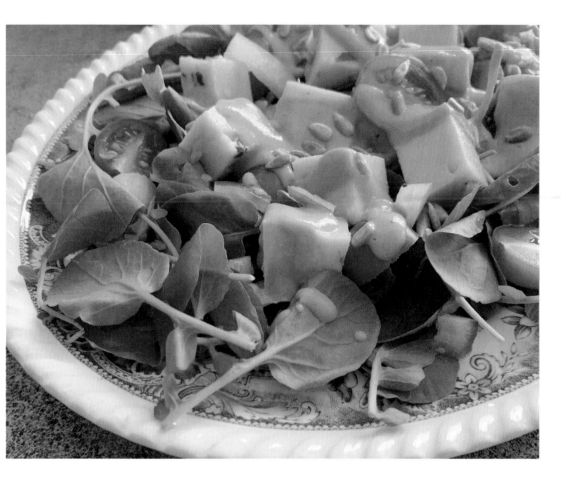

In a small bowl, whisk together sunflower seed butter, lemon juice, coconut aminos, remaining ¼ teaspoon of garlic powder, mustard, and reishi powder. Add water, 1 teaspoon at a time, until dressing reaches your preferred thinness (about 4 teaspoons water).

To assemble individual servings, divide the watercress, tomatoes, bell pepper, and red onion among 4 plates. Using a sharp knife, cut the chilled polenta into 1-inch/2.5 cm cubes and add a handful to each salad. Top with the dressing and sunflower seeds. Leftover polenta keeps for 1 week in the refrigerator; before using, pour off any excess water that pools during storage.

*Omit the reishi if you're pregnant or breastfeeding, and always consult with your doctor before introducing a new functional food into your diet.

141

Jasmine Cacao Brain-Boosting Tonic

Like a grown-up hot chocolate, this energizing drink reverses a workday slump with antioxidant-rich cacao and sophisticated, floral notes of jasmine—an energy-shifting trigger for the parasympathetic nervous system. Lion's mane mushroom increases the production of brain health–supporting nerve growth factor, further enhancing workday focus and flow.

SERVES 1

1 cup/250 ml unsweetened nondairy milk

½ teaspoon loose-leaf jasmine tea

1 tablespoon cacao powder

1 tablespoon pure maple syrup

½ teaspoon lion's mane mushroom powder*

Pour the milk into a saucepan and heat over low heat until warm. Add the remaining ingredients and whisk until incorporated. Warm over low heat for 3 minutes while the jasmine tea steeps. Strain through a fine-mesh sieve into a mug and serve warm.

*Omit the lion's mane if you're pregnant or breastfeeding, and always consult with your doctor before introducing a new functional food into your diet.

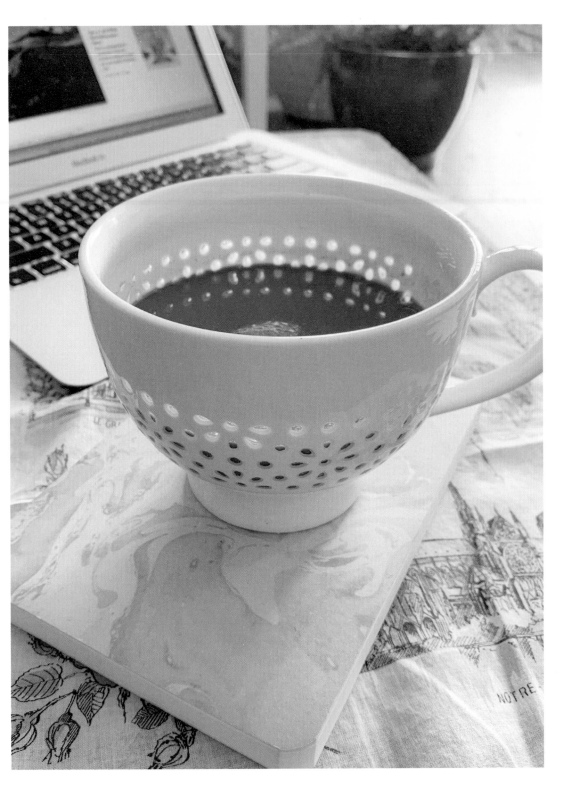

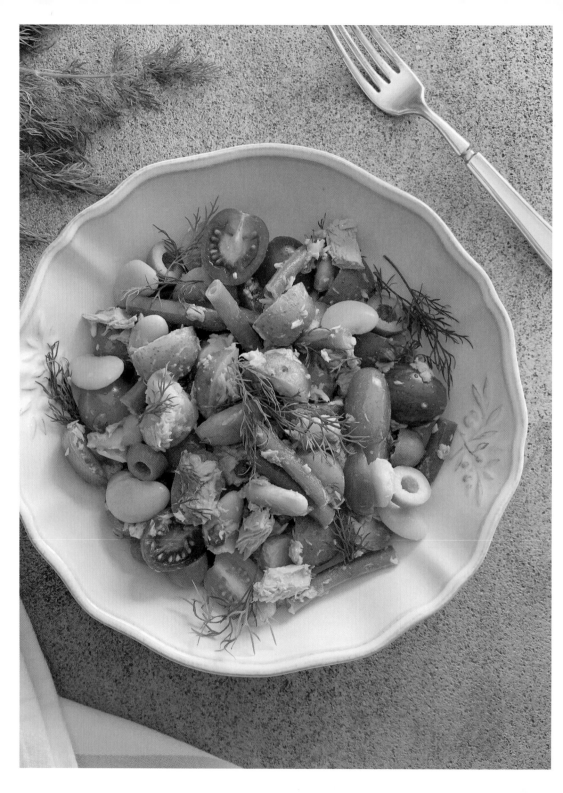

No-Time Niçoise Salad

This infinitely adaptable salad inspires me creatively, delights my palate, and comes together in no time flat—making it a staple on busy workdays. Sub in your favorite beans, pickled veggies, or whatever fresh produce you have on hand to suit your mood and energy when you make it.

SERVES 4

1 pound/450 g organic potatoes, scrubbed and cut into bite-size chunks

8 ounces/230 g green beans, cut into bite-size pieces

1 (15-ounce/440 g) BPA-free can beans (I like cannellini or butter beans), drained and rinsed

2 cups/300 g cherry or grape tomatoes, halved

½ cup/50 g pitted olives, halved

2 tablespoons/20 g capers

1 (5-ounce/142 g) can non-albacore tuna (I like skipjack tuna), drained

2 tablespoons/10 g chopped fresh dill

¼ cup/60 ml olive oil

2 tablespoons/30 ml cider vinegar

2 teaspoons whole-grain mustard

Unrefined salt

Place the potatoes in a pot and cover with 2 inches/5 cm of water. Bring to a boil and simmer for 5 to 6 minutes, or until tender. Use a slotted spoon to remove the potatoes from the water and set aside to cool. Add the green beans to the water, return to a boil, and cook for 5 minutes, or until tender. Drain, rinse with cool water to stop the cooking, and set aside to cool. Meanwhile, in a large serving bowl, combine the beans, tomatoes, olives, capers, tuna, and dill. Once the potatoes and green beans have cooled to the touch, add them to the bowl as well. In a small bowl, whisk together the remaining ingredients, adding salt to taste. Pour the dressing over the salad and stir to combine. Serve immediately.

Sunny Day Seed Crackers

These hearty crackers are portable, convenient fuel that pack an impressive amount of nutrition and flavor. Their combination of nutritional yeast, tamari, and garlic gives them a savory depth that pairs well with so many toppings, including my favorite: goat cheese and fresh herbs.

MAKES 40 CRACKERS

½ cup/85 g flaxseeds, divided

¼ cup/47 g chia seeds

½ cup/68 g raw sunflower seeds, plus more for topping, if desired

½ cup/68 g raw pumpkin seeds

3 tablespoons/20 g nutritional yeast

¼ teaspoon garlic powder

1 cup/250 ml water

3 tablespoons/40 ml low-sodium tamari

Preheat the oven to 350°F/180°C. Line a large baking sheet with parchment paper.

In a high-powered blender or food processor, grind ¼ cup/42 g of the flaxseeds and the chia seeds into a powder. Transfer the powder to a large bowl. Add the sunflower and pumpkin seeds to the blender or food processor and pulse once or twice, just enough to chop the seeds. Add the pulsed seeds, remaining whole flaxseeds, nutritional yeast, and garlic powder to the bowl and stir to combine. Pour the water and tamari over the seed mixture and mix well. Set aside for 5 to 10 minutes to absorb.

Using a spoon or clean, damp fingers, spread the seed mixture on the prepared baking sheet, creating a smooth, thin 16 x 13-inch rectangle that is about ¼ inch thick. Sprinkle the top of the mixture with sunflower seeds, if desired, and gently press them in. Bake for 30 minutes, remove from the oven, and carefully cut into 2 x 3-inch/5 x 7.5 cm crackers on the baking sheet (a pizza cutter works very well here). Flip

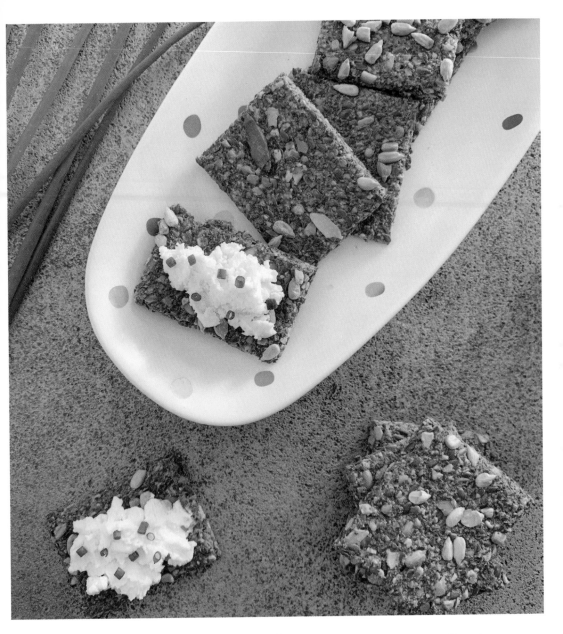

the crackers and return to the oven for 15 minutes more. Remove from the oven and allow to cool on the baking sheet before serving. Store in an airtight container for up to 1 week, or freeze for 2 months.

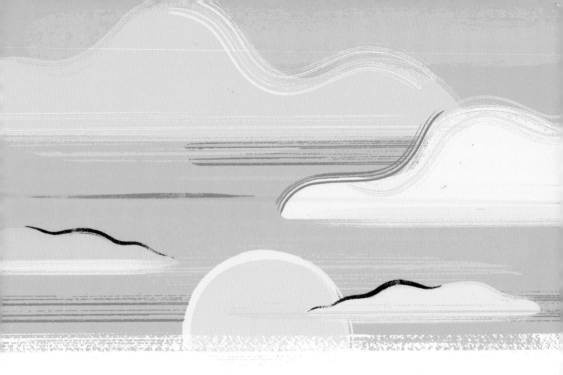

chapter four

Sunset

Sunset is your time to choose joy.

The sun begins to sink, its light casting filters that range from peachy gold to ethereal blue over your world. That fading light conjures everyday magic as the sun reaches its climactic moment on the horizon. It might release laserlike rays from its dipping point as it disappears from view, or electrify the clouds for a fleeting burst of candy-colored purples and pinks that shift in real time, leaving you basking in the afterglow. Other days, it's an almost imperceptible fade until you notice that blackness has crept in. Those are the lights of sunset.

No two sunsets are ever exactly alike, much like the sunset hours of our day. Sunset is a transition time, one that's a pivotal point for your energy. For many of us, it's also the time when we finally retake full control of the narrative of our day. Although you might still have a list of chores and commitments, it's more likely that sunset is the time when you can create more essential moments of joy in your day. You decide what sunset will hold. If your sunset routine has little room for choice, this chapter will give you incentive to take control of your precious sunset hours and guide them to fulfill their energetic potential of joy and self-care.

The best sunset hours are like "choose your own adventure" stories. They're open to daily change, ripe for reinvention, and far more flexible than sunrise or daylight. No matter what your sunset routine, I recommend creating a ritual of a quick energy self-assessment as you transition into sunset hours. This could happen around the time that you're commuting home from work, heading out to dinner with friends, or thinking about what you'll do during the evening hours. Pause and ask yourself, "What's my energy like in this moment?" "Am I holding onto unwanted energy from earlier parts of my day?" and "What does my body need this evening to restore its energetic brightness?" Your responses will differ based on the day you've had so far. Use the answers to guide your sunset hours.

SUNSET ENERGY THEMES

joy · introspection · home spaces · self-care · sounds · comforts · happiness · laughter · gathering · nourishment

REFLECT ON YOUR SUNSET ENERGY

What responsibilities do I have to attend to at this time of day? Can I fully detach from daylight tasks?

How often do I have unscheduled time for play? How do I use that time?

What's the feeling I get from my home environment?

Who else affects my sunset energy? People? Pets?

How much time do I spend with TV or other devices at this time of day?

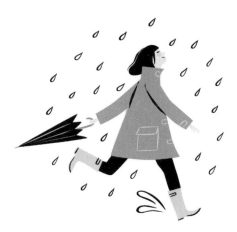

Nature's Energy: Water and Natural Objects

Sunset is the time to connect to the energy of water and its ability to cleanse, refresh, and replenish you. We often literally cleanse at this time of day by washing our hands when we return home, showering, maybe even taking a bath or a swim in the evening to refresh mind and body. Submerging the body in water has well-established associations with cleansing and starting anew, from baptism to baths used to detox and clear unwanted energy to clearing of chakras with water. And symbolically we may cleanse away the day by closing laptops, leaving offices, changing clothes, and shifting our focus from daylight tasks.

I encourage you to make water a sunset symbol that reminds you to replenish your body with pure water as you transition to sunset and drink water again while you prepare dinner or before you dine, since prehydrating your digestive tract can help you better digest and assimilate the nutrients in your food. You might also want to use the sounds of water—trickling, flowing, falling drops, crashing waves—if you need to calm your energy and fill your space with peaceful sounds at this time of day. If you happen to live near a body of water, such as a lake, stream, or ocean, you've probably noticed that spending time there brightens your mood.

Waterside spots are particularly sought after for healing, restoring, and resetting energy, likely because negative ions concentrate in the air around bodies of water (and notably in the air in your bathroom when you shower or bathe). These negative ions have impressive potential to brighten and balance your energy. Negative ions reduce stress on the body, boost mood, (one study found that sitting in a room with a concentration of negative ions for 30 minutes a day was enough to significantly improve symptoms of seasonal affective disorder), heighten alertness by increasing oxygen flow to the brain, and even clear many airborne germs. Positive ions, on the other hand (emitted by computers and appliances, and often concentrated in cities and stuffy offices or homes) can cause sleepiness, headaches, raise stress levels, and even make you more prone to respiratory illness.

Water flows over and around barriers and blockages that get in its way, making it a symbol of persistence, perpetuity, and resilience that I love. Whatever blockages you've encountered so far during this day, find a way to divert your path around them to reach this moment of restoration and replenishment. Use the bright energy that you've built up so far to continue your progress toward your energetic goals of joy, resilience, and feeling lit from within.

Sunset energy also aligns with the varied natural objects that you bring into your home and surroundings—think: plants, crystals, flowers, rocks, feathers, wood, sand, stone, shells, and countless others. Recent study has proven the therapeutic value of natural objects, such as flowers, in reducing anxiety and fatigue and boosting positive feelings, while lowering blood pressure, heart rate, and pain perception. Surrounding yourself with the things that evoke personal joy is the essence of sunset energy, as you'll read ahead. In Chapter 1, we learned that these objects each carry their own vibrations, and together they have the power to influence the four facets of your energy—body, mind, emotions, and spirit. Let your intuition guide you to the objects that feel most replenishing to you in your day.

Top Sunset Energy Drains

※ **No time or space to unwind**

※ **Daylight work that continues through the evening without rest**

※ **A home environment that feels uncomfortable**

※ **An evening meal that doesn't adequately replenish your body after a day of work**

※ **Too much time spent with devices that leave you drained or stressed**

SUNSET ENERGY INFLUENCERS

A big secret to feeling joy in your life every single day is creating it for yourself. Of course, you'll often serendipitously find joy in your day, but to keep your bright energy flowing, it helps immensely to build in joyful moments that you are certain to encounter each day. If you're in a place of struggle, this is even more essential to your journey to ignite your light. Ahead, you'll find specific ways to build joy by looking at the sunset energy influencers that serve as three self-guided opportunities for you to experience joy each day. First, we'll look at the transformative experience of play that's absent from so many of our routines. Then, we'll take note of how we draw energy from our home spaces and the other interiors where we repeatedly gather and spend time—especially during our sunset hours. And, finally, we'll use the energy of music and sound to clear our energy and reinforce pathways of bliss in our brains and bodies. Overall, sunset is your time for joy and self-care, even amid the remaining tasks and to-dos in your day. Claim it and feel its power to light you up!

WILD AND FREE: THE ENERGY OF PLAY AND LAUGHTER

Watch a child at play and you'll witness bright energy in action. Squealing, giggling, risk taking, exploring, discovering, all without awareness of time or duty—that's the energy of play. Watching that playing child may even take you back to a feeling of freedom and lightness whose role in your life has retreated over time. For the sake of beauty, resilience, and joy in your life, this is the moment to welcome that feeling again. **Play is an ideal way to release stagnant, blocked energy, as well as an antidote to the heaviness of life that shakes up your routine, challenges you, and helps you see your world differently.** While we often hear that play is an essential part of child development, we forget that it's just as valuable for adults, who often remove it from their priorities. Adults derive incredible energetic and physical benefits from consciously including play in their daily routines; these are benefits you can see, feel, and lean on when challenges arise.

There are a thousand ways to play, so don't feel as though you need to pull out a board game or initiate a round of tag to experience the energy of play. The only play essential is that you approach your chosen activity with a mindset of openness and discovery. Let time go, live in the moment, and seek only to enjoy yourself. This approach to play takes the complexity out of life, if only for a moment. The more you repeat it, the more time your brain and body spend in that free, simple, and pure state of being—one where you're immersed in bright energy.

Find your favorite forms of play by thinking about experiences that bring you pure joy, or look for ways to involve play in your current routine. Try taking something you already do and add an element of play to it. If you practice yoga, take an aerial yoga class; if you love taking walks, add a scavenger hunt to your next loop around the block; if you are a voracious reader, incorporate some humor books into your stack. If you're still feeling awkward about play, retrace your steps to the types of play that brought you joy at other times in your life. Did you once love coloring, or building sandcastles? Start there.

If needed, schedule in a play break, fifteen minutes at a time, until it feels more natural. While you're playing, remember to consciously take in the feeling of the activity. Allow your joy to sink in, to produce an even stronger shift in your long-term energy. The freedom and lightness of play signal to your brain and your body that life is joyful, and bright energy flows.

Play allows us to shake off the dust that settles over our worldview, especially when we're dealing with complex moments that inevitably come with adult life. The secret is the freedom and the space that your brain and body experience during play. Play gives you the opportunity to think, move, and discover in a fresh, uninhibited way. Unsurprisingly, those who play are more resilient, develop better stress-coping skills, and often even have healthier brains, thanks to the effect of neurogenesis, the development of brain neurons. The act of play boosts brain function by secreting a substance called BDNF that supports the growth of new brain cells. Over time, it improves memory, encourages creativity, and helps you learn and form new brain pathways faster. When you play with others, you deepen bonding and communication, lighting up the

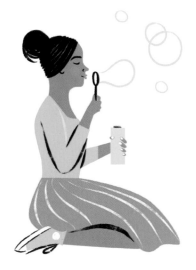

relationship and connection area of energy in your life as well. And did you know that play has beauty benefits? Playfulness has been shown to boost your attractiveness; scientific explanation finds that playfulness signals the presence of attractive, magnetic qualities, including nonaggressiveness, youth, and fertility. And physical play counts as movement and exercise, with a spectrum of physical and energetic benefits. Sunset play is a perfect time to catch up on movement if you were too busy to move your body during the sunrise and daylight portions of your day.

FORGOTTEN HOW TO PLAY?

I know lots of adults who, when they actually sit down to play, find it hard. If play feels unnatural, or you've forgotten how, try these simple practices that support the bright energy of play:

Swing on the swings at a park.

Buy an inexpensive set of watercolors and paint something you like.

Run, roll, or sled down a hill.

Bounce on a trampoline.

Have a water balloon fight.

Doodle.

Learn a new joke.

Jump through a sprinkler.

Go for a bike ride.

Try a new word puzzle or crossword.

Tip: If you're not physically able to do some of these things, start by imagining yourself doing them. Your brain doesn't differentiate between experience and vivid imagination and you'll receive many of the same energy benefits.

Laughing Out Loud

Where there's play, there's likely to be spontaneous laughter. Laughter's role as a healing tool is profound—and it takes effect as soon as you even *anticipate* something funny. One study found that the anticipation of watching a funny film boosted anti-inflammatory beta endorphins by 27 percent and lowered cortisol by 39 percent even before the laughs began. That's reason enough to find something, or someone, that makes you laugh and keep it close! Laughter has the unique ability to instantly shift dim energy and bring lightness to the darkest of situations. It's bonding and it's contagious—think of the energy exchange happening when you're next to someone who's laughing—making it hard to resist.

Why does laughter feel healing on so many levels? Laughter tells your brain to restrict the stress hormone cortisol, even as it releases endorphins that relieve physical, emotional, and psychological pain. It reduces inflammation (a major boon to clear, luminous skin and balanced hormones), boosts your immune system by increasing powerful defense cells called lymphocytes, and helps clear dim energy to make room for light. It's even been shown to reduce serious symptoms of disease, such as pain and depression.

Like play, laughter is restorative; it counters the depletion and overwhelm that so many of us feel in our daily routines. It momentarily takes you out of time and space, to a place where there is only joy. When you feel that joy, your body releases a cocktail of brain chemicals. Those compounds, and your brain chemistry at large, influence your blood chemistry too, unleashing a whole-body effect on the four facets of your energy. Further effects of joy are as diverse as faster wound healing and recovery from illness, better digestion and metabolism, and even a longer life span. By consciously focusing on joy, you're training your brain to fully experience a state of happiness that is sometimes lost or diminished when we're dealing with pain or trauma, or simply not feeling our best. Consciously choosing joy—by playing and laughing even when those activities feel hard—is one of the best tools to lift yourself up out of the darkest times. And when you come through it surrounded by joy, you'll create beauty in the entire experience.

The joy that comes from play and laughter is such a positive experience for the brain that it allows you to see broadened possibilities, which in turn make it more likely that you'll develop new skills. Scientific study has found that positive emotions, such as happiness, release neurotransmitters that boost memory and ability to learn. And learning and developing new skills leads to more positive experiences, and then to more happiness, and the positive cycle continues. Joy itself is invigorating to the human mind and nourishing to the four facets of your energy. It's a worthy pursuit at any time of the day, but you may find it especially abundant during the sunset hours.

THE GAMIFICATION OF TECH

The closest that many adults get to play these days is in a smartphone game. And wow, are they addictive, designed to readily release the four primary happiness-influencing brain chemicals: dopamine, oxytocin, serotonin, and endorphins. And it's not just games that are being designed with brain chemicals in mind; just about everything tech-related aims to produce feel-good brain chemicals with the goal of keeping you coming back again and again—one clever way to create loyal customers. Are these experiences really boosting your joy in the long run? And are they truly channeling the bright energy that ignites your light? Take a step back from your regular tech interactions so you can judge for yourself. And aim to put down your phone or tablet and play in a way that creates your own joy if it's been a while.

My biggest play energy shift came when:
I treated play like a valuable part of my healing process,
rather than a distraction from my to-do list.

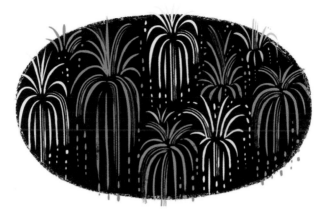

PLAY ENERGY IN PRACTICE: ACUPUNCTURE

The concept of acupuncture—sticking tiny, hair-width needles into the skin to support energy flow—doesn't initially call to mind fun or playfulness for most of us. But look closer: the universally balancing, energy-freeing effects of acupuncture look a lot like those of the joyful state that results from laughter and play. Like joy, acupuncture releases endorphins that give the body a natural high that dulls pain and can even make us feel giddy.

Some of my most surprisingly blissed-out moments have caught me, unexpectedly, after an acupuncture session, when those endorphins were flooding my brain. During the lows of chronic illness, I recall one particular acupuncture treatment that felt as if it set off blissful fireworks in my brain. If you are having difficulty shifting your energy, are struggling with illness or imbalance, or are just having trouble feeling bliss from play and laughter at this time, the powerful effect of circulating energy during acupuncture treatment is a must-try.

So, how does acupuncture work? Acupuncture says that your energy, or qi, flows through the body along meridian pathways, which form a map of over two thousand acupoints located just below the surface of your skin. Your practitioner will insert thin needles into your skin at points

159

that correspond to your unique needs. Your only job is to relax, visualize energy flowing, and let the blissed-out feeling grow. Not only does acupuncture have the ability to decrease pain and increase nitric oxide, a gas that improves circulation (giving you a radiant afterglow), it is very likely to uplift you in the process. A UK study found that acupuncture had a remarkably positive effect on depression, producing a reduction in symptoms that lasted for three months after treatment. Another study found that a form of acupuncture called electroacupuncture (in which the acupuncture needles carry a mild electric current) was just as effective at reducing symptoms of depression as treatment with prescription Prozac. And overall, acupuncture is known for its feel-good effects that can bring about a feeling of balance and homeostasis that will leave you amazed at the impact of your energy flow.

If you're new to the practice, I encourage you to try a series of acupuncture sessions (a few in short sequence often have a cumulative effect and may be more likely to produce big results). Acupuncture is a valuable tool that can help you release energy blocks and create a euphoric sense of joy and well-being that comes from uninhibited energy flow in the body.

⩾ Energy Booster ⩽

Try bringing extra childlike joy into your home by filling it with rainbows. Inexpensive crystal window films (find them online) are an easy way to filter incoming light into spectacular rainbow patterns on your home walls. Apply them to your west-facing windows to bring a joyful light show into your home space and increase the bright energy around you during the sunset hours!

EMINÉ'S SUNSET

NAME: Eminé Rushton

WHAT TO KNOW ABOUT ME:
I'm an author and wellbeing writer, a holistic facialist and student of nature, as well as a mama of two amazing, noisy, hilarious girls.

THE SUNSET HOURS OF MY DAY ARE USUALLY:
Savored.

MY ESSENTIALS FOR THE BEST SUNSET ENERGY:
A mug of deep, dark cacao; a flickering candle; a book; a rose and jasmine bath—these restore my energy to no end.

FAVORITE WAY TO FUEL MY BODY DURING SUNSET HOURS:
A beautiful, still, silent bath. Sometimes I can stay in the tub for over an hour. Sinking into the bath, I almost hold my breath so as not to pierce the stillness of it all. I love the peaceful cocoon afforded us when we are underwater.

SUNSET ENERGY INFLUENCERS AFFECT MY PERSONAL ENERGY MOST IN THE AREA OF:
Play and laughter. My evening is filled with my kids' raucous laughter and antics, and I love that dichotomy between their energetic explosions and then, once they're in bed, my own inward, silent contemplation. During these hours, I keep my technology in another room, in order to be fully present with my kids. There's a sacredness to just being with your loved ones, with nothing at all to distract you—listening, conversing, sharing, seeing. My kids are always much calmer at bedtime when they've had this uninterrupted time with me, and I too am much calmer with my mind in one place only.

THE LIGHT AROUND YOU:
THE ENERGY OF INTERIOR SPACES

It's pretty overwhelming to think of all of the spaces you've spent time in over the years: classrooms, offices, hotel rooms, airports, homes, restaurants, to name only a few. At times it's even a challenge to keep track of the places you visit during a single day. Yet I bet you can recall—even superficially—how most of those spaces made you feel. You may not have set foot in a particular space for years; the space may exist at present only in your memory, yet you can call to mind how its energy affected you while you were there. This is the influential energy of interior spaces.

We know inherently that the interior spaces we spend time in impact us. But we're at a loss to change most of the spaces we visit, even if we have strong feelings about their energetic effects. Some, like offices or schools, we spend time in to fulfill duties or meet goals. Others, like museums or spas, we visit because we enjoy the activities that take place there. But your home is unique. You actually have the power to shape the place, or places, that you call home into an environment that reflects and restores your energy and ignites your light.

When you enter your home, it's as if your energy field suddenly expands to envelop everything within its walls. Your home space is a part of your world in such a personal way that at times it feels like an extension of your inner self. So,

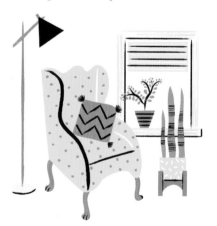

what does your ideal energetic home look like? And what should every energetically bright home space contain? I urge you to shrug off any pressure you feel to curate your home according to a particular decorating style or formula. Creating a space that ignites your light whenever you spend time there starts with simply bringing in more of what you love. A thing of beauty itself serves

162

your body in a positive way. When you look at something that brings you feelings of joy, balance, and well-being, this experience benefits all four facets of your energy. If you give yourself only one mission from this section, make it this: **find beautiful things, bring them into your home, feel gratitude and joy from them, and watch how that changes you and your space.** You might opt for rocks or plants, plush pillows, vivid artwork, or a group of beloved friends or family. Although wildly different, each of these wields power over the energy of your home space.

Your Energetic Home

Your energy comes to life within the walls of your home. Your home reflects your personal energy, and in turn its energy reflects back to you and all those who enter. From the early morning thoughts you have in your bed to the space where you curl up with a book in the evening, your home serves as both an inner retreat and a material embodiment of you and your thoughts, values, and choices. Establishing the energy you want at home grounds you during the time you spend there; you hold onto that energy as you venture out into the world and into varied spaces and influences across your day.

Do you know the energy of your home? Start here to create a clear energetic vision for your space:

Define the role that you want your home space to have in your life. Maybe it serves as a retreat from the demands of the outside world, an appealing gathering place for your family, the sophisticated apartment of your dreams, or a blank slate where you can express your creativity whenever you spend time there. If your home space has more than one purpose, list them all.

As you get clear on the key role of your home, it's also helpful to consider the energy of your daylight hours and reflect on the ways that the energy of your home can help you maintain balance. If you spend the day in a raucous elementary school classroom, perhaps you'd like your home space to be minimalist and serene. If your daylight hours are full of computer coding, maybe you keep most of your home space screen-free. You might aim for a yin/yang balance between daylight and sunset activities.

Choose one or two words that describe how you want your home space to feel. What words embody the energy you want from your home? Are there specific textures, colors, or objects that you associate with these words?

Sometimes it's hard to describe the energy you want, but you know it when you feel it. After more than a decade of renting apartments, it took me and my husband nine months of searching to find a home with the right energy. We both felt it as soon as we entered the space. This home instantly conveyed a feeling of serenity, healing, and light that we so needed while I was in the depths of chronic illness. Since then, this home—our home—has become such a healing place for me, one that I derive so much joy and bright energy from!

When it comes to creating your ideal energetic home space, you make the rules. But I do find these six guidelines to be especially valuable as you design a space that ignites your light:

6 ESSENTIALS FOR YOUR
BEST HOME ENERGY

1) Create a dedicated spot where you can recharge. Choose a restorative spot within your space where you feel happy, peaceful, and inspired. Add objects that convey energy and meaning to you. For me, it's my sunroom, where I can flood myself with natural light no matter what the season. It's filled with green plants and a few big chairs that are conducive to reading, meditating, writing, or napping.

2) Cut down or eliminate energy drains. Take stock of your surroundings in each new season and clean out or remove what no longer serves you. Toss expired food from the refrigerator, tackle the pile of clothes in your bedroom, and eliminate unwanted clutter—a process that may take time.

3) Bring nature inside. Remember all of those grounding, stabilizing effects of nature? You can take them with you—right inside your home. I love natural objects that also convey emotions and memories of a particular place or person.

4) Set out reminders of your values and goals. A devotional on your bedside table, a pretty water filter on your countertop, a sign IGNITE YOUR LIGHT posted near your keys so you see it as you walk out the door—these types of items help you stay connected to your desired energy.

5) Keep a few purely indulgent objects, for the purpose of sheer joy or self-care for you or your family. You can't avoid dim energy outside of your home, but you *can* make your home space one of overwhelming comfort and light.

6) If possible, make your home a place that supports you in optimizing the other energy influencers in your life: people, movement, creativity, nourishment, and so on. You might include a dedicated space for working out, an easel where you can paint when inspiration strikes, an inviting living room for loved ones to gather in, or a color-coded closet for your morning preparation routine.

The message here is not that there's one particular way to create your space; rather, that you should carefully consider the effect that your home space (as well as any space you spend ample time in) has on your energy. Let your energy guide you to places, objects, colors, and textures you love, without needing a reason. It's an exercise in energy awareness. Home organizing approaches, such as feng shui and KonMari, offer abundant inspiration, but know that they might not align with your desires. One example: feng shui principles warn against cacti in your home, claiming that their spikes create negative energy. I'm not convinced!

Interior Energy Features: DECO

Keep these four energy features in mind as you fine-tune the energy of your home space. The acronym DECO—décor, environment, color, order—can help you remember to assess how each feature influences in your space.

DÉCOR: *objects and their meaning*

ENVIRONMENT: *scent, temperature, sound, and light*

COLOR: *the visible hues in your space*

ORDER: *structure, arrangement, and flow*

D: DÉCOR

Every object has energy—this you know. So, what makes the energy of one preferable to another? The answer is you. Simply put, what you give energy and meaning to takes on bright, healing energetic properties. I strongly believe that it doesn't matter whether you're into crystals or flowers, or you are drawn to birds or butterflies, or you derive energy from old family photographs—there is no limit to the type of objects that shift our energy and help us strengthen our experience of health and beauty. You've already seen that people, places, thoughts, and foods carry a similar energetic influence. Your goal is to reflect on your life, your personal needs, and bring in more of the objects, people, ideas, and so on that light you up—whether or not they are the same objects chosen by others. In my home, my sacred objects include a simple beaded bracelet made by my son, a print that was displayed at my wedding, lamps that used to light my grandparents' home, and a conch shell that I found on a particularly memorable day at the beach. Looking at them floods my body with joy, gratitude, and a surge of healing energy.

CRYSTALS AND YOUR ENERGY

A thing of beauty is a true joy—and crystals have to be one of the most beautiful gifts of nature. Crystals have been prized for centuries for their energetic influence, and this perspective continues to dominate in present day. But I don't believe that crystals are a necessity for an ideal energetic home space. It's much more important, and influential to your energy, that you fill your space with objects to which you have an elevated emotional connection: joy, happiness, security, and comfort are some of the feelings you want to evoke. I have a few crystals that I love because they bring the beauty of nature into my home—another valuable goal. But it's the feeling they convey, not the material itself, that possesses the most healing power for me. Whatever items you choose to support beauty, resilience, and joy in your life, spend time visualizing their brightening effect on your body to reinforce their power. And, of course, treat them with care. Any object that is precious and lovingly cared for will possess inherent healing potential.

E: ENVIRONMENT

Knowing how deeply your senses affect your energy, it follows that the sights, smells, feels, and sounds of your home environment also influence your light. Think about what makes a space feel good to you—is it a particular scent? A comfortable temperature? A certain level of light? **Activating your senses in a way that is pleasing and uplifting starts a chain reaction in your body that immediately shifts your energy and your biology.** Inside your home, you can support this effect by crafting an environment that brings you joy. Don't over-look the energy-shifting power of aromas, from a cozy dinner on the stove, to the fresh-cut grass wafting in the window, to your favorite essential oils in a diffuser. Two excellent essential oils for shifting energy are *Melissa* (also known as lemon balm), called the "oil of light," and Roman chamomile, dubbed the "oil of spiritual purpose." Try diffusing them in combination during the sunset hours—or choose your own favorites.

C: COLOR

At Sunrise, you learned about the energy of colors in your wardrobe; much of the same information can be applied to the colors you use in your home. Recall that each color has its own vibration, from violet (the color with the highest vibration) in reverse rainbow order down to red (which has the lowest vibra-tion). Refer to pages 81–82 for popular interpretations of color meaning and energy that you can apply to your home. Remember that each of the seven main colors are also associated with one of the body's chakras, the primary energy centers of the body. Supporting a particular chakra can involve bringing more of that color into your environment.

O: ORDER

Regardless of the personal style that creates visual and energetic harmony for you, it helps to step back and take a look at the larger order of your home reflected by its structure, arrangement, and flow. It could be that a change in the order of your home would produce an even bigger energetic shift than different colors or décor ever could. If you're a homeowner, ask yourself whether there are larger changes you could make to help the energy of your home to match your goals. Adding bigger windows, installing a cozy fireplace, opening up a space, or designing an addition—what would give your home new energetic life? And how could you streamline or rearrange the flow of your home to better sup-port your energy and goals?

When Past Becomes Present

Think about the three most valued objects you own. I bet that most, if not all, have ties to the past. Some of my most precious possessions once belonged to beloved relatives who have passed. They are few and carefully selected because they evoke specific memories of joy or gratitude. But what happens if relics from the past (yours or someone else's) bring up dim or conflicting energy for you? Or if objects are passed down to you, but you simply don't enjoy them? Give yourself the opportunity to reflect honestly on whether an object supports your home's bright energy or you merely feel obligated to maintain it.

If an object's energy doesn't match your own, resolve to let it go. You might want to create a box, or boxes, of special mementos that you enjoy looking through on occasion, and free yourself from the rest. Perhaps you take time to look through them and reflect as you enter a new phase—a new year, a new age, a new job, a new home—or find yourself needing guidance on a decision. Periodically check in with your space to see whether any of the past objects in your home feel out of place with your desired energy in the present.

While you're at it, make sure that your surroundings, or the objects inside them, don't steal energy. Although you can find tremendous joy in collections or maximalist decor, you probably notice that possessions influence both your personal and your metabolic energy, as they take time, thought, and effort to maintain. Clutter can be a tremendous energy drain when the necessary maintenance of objects requires time and effort that could be freed up for creativity, pleasure, and unscheduled time. There's no rule that says you need to live in a minimalist space; simply aim to avoid the kind of clutter that drains you. Consciously curate a space that energizes you and you'll see and feel more lightness in your life.

My biggest interiors energy shift came when:
I stopped trying to fill space in my new home, and instead removed things that didn't have meaning or value to me.

INTERIORS ENERGY IN PRACTICE:
CLEARING THE AIR

Smudging is a beautiful energy cleansing ritual that has deep roots in indigenous American ceremonies used to cleanse or bless a person or place. If you're new to the concept, smudging is often practiced today by burning bundled sage, palo santo, or incense to clear energy in a space, or around your body. This ritual can be as simple as carrying the smoking embers of your chosen smudging material through a space (remember to open the windows to let in fresh air while you smudge), or can involve various prayers or incantations and take on a specific order or directions. You might choose to practice this ritual when you move into a new home, after meditation, or when you feel like the energy in your space needs shifting. But if this ritual doesn't speak to you, try another method of clearing the air in your home. Any time you change the scent, light, air, or even the contents of your home, you inherently shift its energy.

Diffusing essential oils is another powerful way to change the energy of a space while delivering the secondary benefits of killing many airborne germs. And simply opening windows and doors to let fresh air enter can have the very real benefit of bringing more calming negative ions into your home space.

⪢ Energy Booster ⪡

So many of the important objects in our lives are now digital, meaning we don't actually see them or interact with them regularly. Take time to print digital photographs, to bring your virtual vision board to life, and to make in-person connections to those with whom you network on social media.

GOOD VIBRATIONS: THE ENERGY OF SOUND AND MUSIC

What does the sunset of your day sound like? Maybe you flip on your favorite playlist during your commute home, step into the buzz of a packed restaurant where you'll meet friends for dinner, laugh at the squeals of children playing at the park while you walk your dog, or turn on a soothing symphony as you slip out of your work clothes at home. In this moment, the sounds that hit your ears have a profound effect on your energy. It's likely that you've been outputting great amounts of physical and cognitive energy to perform during your daylight hours, and the sounds that fill the sunset of your day can become valuable tools to create a restorative, uplifting energy shift exactly when you need it.

Sound, like our own energy, takes the form of vibration. **The vibrations generated by words, music, and other sounds are our primary forms of communication; they are not only heard, they can be felt.** The energy of bodies and sounds are similar in that they both vibrate at specific frequencies and their vibrations transmit waves. You'll recall that our own energetic vibrations extend at least throughout the human energy field, or biofield, that surrounds the body. Sound waves can travel even farther, as they move readily through air and water. As sound waves travel to your ear, they vibrate your eardrum and the fluid in your inner ear, becoming electrical signals that send a dynamic message to your brain and create your experience of that sound.

Using specific frequencies of sound, we can actually shift our brain waves to put ourselves into brain states that encourage focus, relaxation, or sleep, to name a few. This process, called brain wave entrainment and often referred to as binaural beats, involves playing slightly different frequencies in each ear, which leads the brain to tune into a unique third frequency that's between the two you hear. Your brain wave patterns sync with whichever frequency you perceive. An alpha brain wave pattern, for example, creates the slower brain wave often produced by meditation, whereas theta results in a pattern of deep relaxation, and delta is associated with deep sleep. A review of twenty studies on brain wave entrainment found it to be effective for relieving stress, pain, headaches, and even PMS. Using headphones, you can listen to binaural beats alone, or play them under other types of music (some frequencies are so low that you don't actually notice them). Instruments like singing bowls create them naturally. As you listen, you change the energy of your brain and body with sound.

The Sound of Music

Think of the last time you had a front row seat to live music. The vibrations of sound coming from the playing instruments probably produced a palpable buzzing throughout your body (and the bodies of others, since listening to live music actually syncs the brain rhythms of concertgoers). Now imagine that those vibrations were not only pleasing to your ears and your brain, but actually supported the beauty and health of your entire body. In this case, imagination and reality overlap. We already know that music can slow your breathing and heart rate, reduce blood pressure, and strengthen your immune system (some music, that is—different styles produce different effects). And we've begun to learn that sound vibrations have healing, balancing effects on our cells. Brain imaging has shown that music stimulates the pleasure centers of the brain, resulting in the release of the feel-good neurotransmitters dopamine, oxytocin, serotonin, and the like. We get a greater release of neurotransmitters from the songs we enjoy most, which often solidifies our musical tastes.

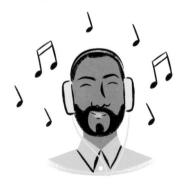

Music has also been shown to light up brain circuits related to the anticipation of reward and surprise. You're in good company if you find that the music you listened to between the ages of 12 and 24 has particular influence over the energy of your body. The reason appears to be that during adolescence and early adulthood our brains undergo rapid development, and the music of that period in our lives often becomes wired to strong, formative emotions and experiences.

I'm always amazed at the ability of sound, especially music, to stir up emotions in my body in mere seconds. When three notes of a familiar song can produce a surge of adrenaline that makes you want to jump out of your seat and dance, or a wave of memory that makes your eyes well with tears, there's no question about the energetic influence of sound.

Through music's ability to activate mirror cells in the brain, you can also experience (or at least glimpse) emotional states conveyed by particular songs. Like play, music takes us out of the present and into a place where time and space are fluid, an ability that's useful in times of emotional or physical stress. Just think of the last time your workout playlist helped you transcend tiredness and run a little faster or farther.

Sound Healing

While it's easy to notice a physical and emotional response to sound vibrations, multiple studies now suggest that the body could even have a specific vibrational bioinformation regulation system that influences us down to the cellular and genetic levels. Further exploration into this possible system could lead to the use of sound and music to produce specific healing effects on the body, from restoring a state of balance to influencing cell regeneration. Because we already know that thoughts, emotions, and beliefs can produce profound changes within the body, it follows that the deep surges of emotion produced by sound and music could also be used to influence our gene expression, healing, and the overall aging process of our bodies.

The idea that vibrations can communicate healing information to the body is the foundation of a practice called sound healing, or vibrational medicine. Sound healing can involve the use of voice, or a range of vibration-producing instruments, including metal or crystal bowls (called singing bowls), tuning forks, chimes, and drums, to produce healing vibrations. I've personally found that certain sound vibrations produce an effect that feels like a gentle, soul-soothing massage, one that envelops my body and can even put it into a state of deep relaxation, right on the edge of sleep yet still aware. Imagine sound waves washing over your body like waves of ocean water and you'll have an idea of what it feels like to experience this energetically soothing practice. The effect feels deep enough to impact me at a cellular level, one of the touted effects of sound healing. And we know that anything that shifts energy to create a state of relaxation in the body and break the mind from a cycle of stress supports health and slows cellular aging. Already one scientific study has demonstrated that hearing singing bowls before meditation leads to lower blood pressure and heart rate, compared to sitting in silence.

The body itself has a rhythm that some compare to music; think of the rhythmic behavior of the heart, breath, and brain, which closely relate to our thoughts and emotions. You can feel sound change the current state of your body. Going further, traditional Chinese Medicine links the five elements— earth, water, metal, fire, and wood—to five specific notes that are believed to influence and support the healthy function of particular organs. Clinical studies have found evidence that music using these five notes significantly decreases depression and cortisol levels, and even improves quality of life for cancer patients. I encourage you to use music and sound to influence your personal energy during the sunset hours and beyond. At this time of day you might crave a euphoric release, quiet calm, or a roaring adrenaline boost.

My biggest sound energy shift came when:
I started using music as a tool to flood my brain with joy in
support of healing.

MUSIC AND SOUND ENERGY
IN PRACTICE: HUM ALONG

You've done it while folding laundry, driving, or showering—especially when there's a catchy melody stuck in your head. Now there's reason to make humming, singing, or chanting a regular part of your energetic day. And the great news: you don't need to be a veteran performer or a karaoke superstar to shift your energy with a song. The vibration coming from your vocal cords when you sing, hum, or chant permeates your body like an energy-shifting wave. And while each of these practices has been found to have slightly different benefits, they all improve immune function, shift and clear blocked energy, relax the body, and boost moods—a list of pros that's well paired with the sunset hours of your day.

Your energy will benefit from simply incorporating any one (or all!) of these vocal practices into your day; no need to study up on technique. If chanting feels unfamiliar, simply think of it as a mix of singing and humming, and start by chanting the word *om* on one extended note. If you enjoy the practice, create your own soothing chants with whatever words speak to you. As you sing, hum, or chant, pay attention to the vibration you create, and the way it feels in your body. You'll notice that you'll feel vibrations resonate in your chest or your nasal passages and head as you lower or raise the tone. Pick one that feels good to you today.

If you're curious or want to take your energy practices to the next level, one specific humming practice called brahmari pranayama has exciting benefits. Humming, and particularly the brahmari pranayama technique, releases nitric oxide into the body, leading to a boost in oxygen delivery and energy production, increased antioxidant production, lowered blood pressure, and improved immunity. The vibration produced by humming has also been shown to help keep your sinuses healthy.

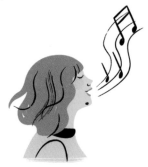

To perform this specific breath-guided humming practice, you traditionally use your thumbs to cover your ears and let your fingers rest on your forehead, atop your eyes. Breathe in deeply through your nose, drop your chin to your chest, and release your breath in a hum. You feel the vibration much more fully when your ears are covered than when they're open. You can play around with the exact tone of your hum, raising or lowering it to find a place where it resonates most fully in your body. Feel the soothing effect of the vibration as it spreads over you. When you've released all of your air, raise your head (keeping your hands in place), take another deep breath through your nose, and drop your chin to your chest to release another long hum. Try repeating this sequence several times, noticing how it shifts your energy and acts like a gentle massage.

Studies suggest that ten minutes of this practice improves cognitive function, while Ayurvedic tradition says that it helps connect your head to your heart and release mental and emotional blocks. As you create more of these soothing, uplifting sounds with your own voice, imagine them shifting and clearing what doesn't serve you. Isn't it amazing to discover new healing, energy-raising practices that are both easy and joyful?

⋟ Energy Booster ⋞

And then there's silence. The absence of sound and vibration, silence is in its own way deeply restorative and healing to the brain and body. When silence feels best, know that giving your body that noise-free time is also restorative to your energy and balancing to the body and mind. Don't be afraid to turn off the music and listen to your breath when you feel quiet calling.

More Ways to Feel the Energy of Sunset

☀ Watch the sun sink into the horizon as you feel yourself disconnect from the unwanted energy sources that are lingering from your day.

☀ If you can, put your devices to "bed" during the sunset hours, and give yourself time to play, wind down, and connect screen-free.

☀ Take a moment to find an object in your home that brings you joy, and remember why you love it so much.

☀ Create your own sunset playlist to produce your desired energy during this part of your day.

RECIPES TO NOURISH YOUR SUNSET ENERGY

Sunset foods are restorative and nourishing, at a time of day when we may gather with families or friends to share a meal. The best encourage experimentation and discovery in the kitchen, so opt for foods that engage the senses with their sights, sounds, and smells. Your sunset recipe repertoire should include main dishes that are easy and nourishing when time is short, and that further healing and self-care as part of a beautiful sit-down meal. Probiotic, fermented food supports good moods and production of happiness-boosting serotonin in the digestive tract, so be creative and top your dishes with pickled veggies, sauerkraut, or probiotic dressings. Above all, let your sunset meals support the playful, joyful feel of this time of day.

Ideal foods for sunset energy:
fermented food; magnesium-rich leafy greens, raw seeds, and dark chocolate; complex carbs, like sweet potatoes and quinoa

Sunset Chill Cocktail

Reach for this cocktail to find your natural chill during the sunset hours. Lemon balm is a beautifully aromatic herb that lowers stress and anxiety, boosts brain function, and helps you digest optimally. It makes a great addition to your herb garden, but if needed, you can substitute mint leaves.

SERVES 6 TO 8

½ cup/190 ml raw honey

½ cup/125 ml water

1 cup/30 g packed fresh lemon balm leaves, plus more for garnish

1 (2-inch/5 cm) piece fresh ginger, sliced

3 to 4 limes

Carbonated water

In a saucepan, combine the honey and water and warm over low heat until the honey dissolves. Add the lemon balm leaves and ginger and stir to coat, pressing down leaves with your spoon for several minutes until they wilt into the liquid (raise the heat slightly, if needed). Remove from the heat, cover, and chill in the refrigerator for 2 hours or overnight. Strain the syrup through a fine-mesh sieve, pressing the lemon balm leaves and ginger with the back of your spoon.

To assemble each cocktail, fill your glass with ice and combine 2 tablespoons/30 ml of the syrup and 1 tablespoon of freshly squeezed lime juice, and top with carbonated water. Garnish with fresh lemon balm leaves and lime slices.

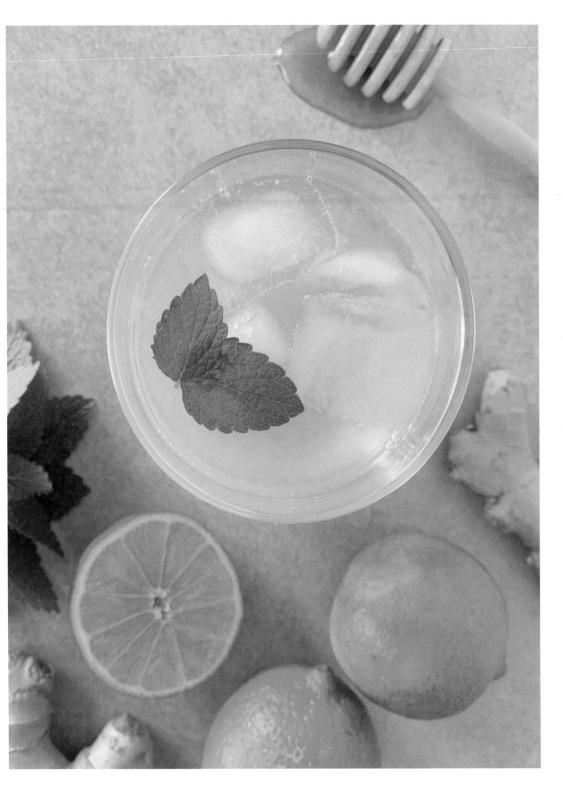

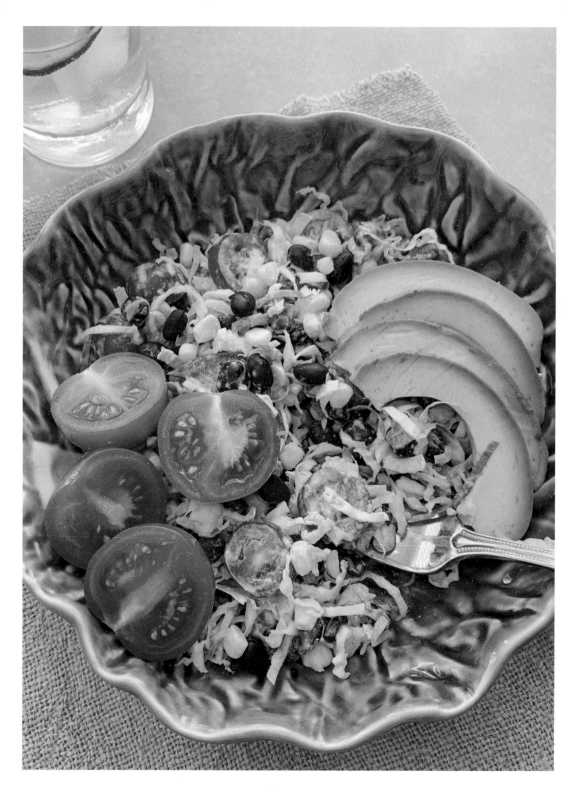

Cashew Jalapeño Beans and Greens Bowl

Taco flavors are a perpetual crowd-pleaser in my home, so the energy of this dish is fun and festive whenever I make it. Creamy cashew tones down the jalapeño so just a hint of heat remains, with plenty of fresh crunch from the shredded Brussels sprouts.

SERVES 4

½ cup/65 g raw cashews

½ cup/120 ml water

2 medium-size jalapeño peppers, seeds and membranes removed

2 tablespoons/30 ml freshly squeezed lemon juice

Scant ¼ teaspoon unrefined salt

12 ounces/340 g Brussels sprouts, finely shredded

1 (15-ounce/440 g) BPA-free can black beans, drained and rinsed

1½ cups/200 g corn kernels

3 cups/450 g cherry tomatoes, halved

2 scallions, finely sliced

1 ripe avocado, pitted, peeled and sliced

In a high-powered blender, combine the cashews, water, jalapeños, lemon juice, and salt until smooth. Set aside. In a large bowl, mix together the shredded Brussels sprouts, beans, corn, tomatoes, and scallions. Add the dressing and toss to coat. Divide into 4 servings and top each with ¼ sliced avocado.

Miso Lime Marinated Lentils

These tangy-sweet lentils make a satisfying side with enough protein to double as a main course. This recipe can be made ahead of time; just toss in the red cabbage at the last minute to keep it crunchy. Edible flowers bring bright energy to every serving, so they're well worth the effort to seek out!

SERVES 4

1 cup/220 g dried French green lentils, rinsed and drained

3 garlic cloves, peeled

4 cups/1 L water

¼ cup/60 ml olive oil

¼ cup/60 ml freshly squeezed lime juice (from about 2 limes)

1½ teaspoons white miso paste

1 teaspoon apple cider vinegar

2 cups/240 g finely shredded purple cabbage

Handful of fresh chives, chopped

Edible flowers (optional—try chive blossoms or nasturtium)

Combine the lentils, garlic, and water in a medium pot and bring to a boil over high heat. Lower the heat to low and simmer about 15 minutes, or until the lentils are tender. Drain well and transfer to a serving bowl. Remove the garlic cloves, mash, and return to the bowl.

While the lentils cook, whisk together the olive oil, lime juice, miso, and vinegar to make the marinade. Pour the marinade over the warm lentils, stirring to coat well. Stir in the cabbage and chives. Top with edible flowers (if using) and serve.

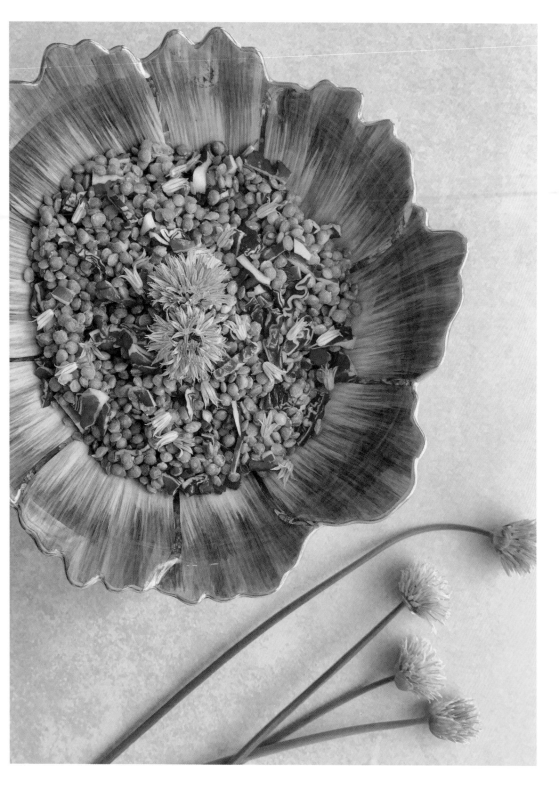

Savory Chickpea Pancake with Spinach and Sun-Dried Tomato

Whipping up pancakes is an act that feels fun and celebratory, so why save that energy for breakfast alone? These savory pancakes are packed with hidden protein from chickpea flour, and they're brightened with a mountain of fresh greens and veggies that gets tied together with a classic vinaigrette. Pair this one with the Sunset Chill Cocktail (page 178), or your favorite evening sip.

SERVES 4

⅓ cup/40 g finely chopped red onion

¼ cup/60 ml red wine vinegar

½ cup/75 g chickpea flour

½ cup/70 g gluten-free flour blend (I like Bob's Red Mill 1-to-1)

1 tablespoon plus 1 teaspoon nutritional yeast

½ teaspoon dried oregano

Unrefined salt

¼ cup plus 2 tablespoons/90 ml olive oil

¼ cup/40 g pitted olives, chopped

Scant ¼ cup/25 g sun-dried tomatoes, finely chopped

1½ cups/380 ml water

4 handfuls organic spinach

¾ cup/130 g chopped tomato

Shelled hemp seeds

In a small bowl, combine the red onion and vinegar and set aside to marinate.

In a medium bowl, combine the chickpea and gluten-free flours, nutritional yeast, oregano, and ¼ teaspoon of the salt. Add 2 tablespoons/30 ml of the olive oil, half of the chopped olives, the sun-dried tomatoes and water, and whisk thoroughly.

Heat a skillet or nonstick pan over medium-low heat and add ½ cup/ 120 ml of the pancake batter. Cook for about 3 minutes, or until golden brown on the first side. Flip and cook

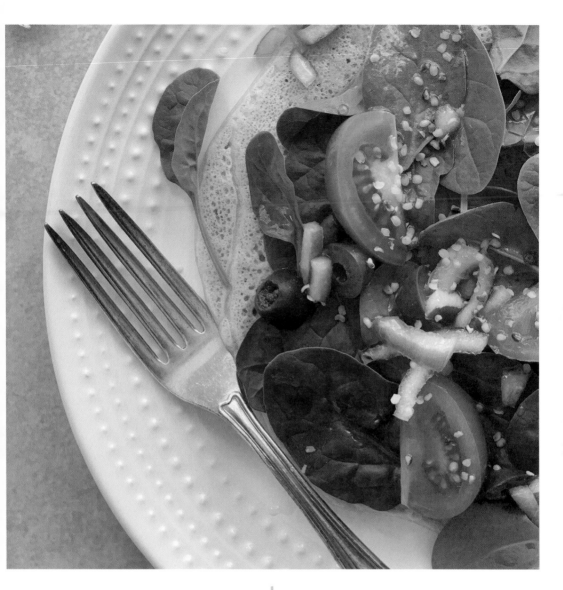

the other side, 1 minute more. Repeat until all 4 pancakes are cooked.

Plate each pancake, top with a handful of spinach, and divide the tomatoes and remaining olives among the plates.

Whisk the remaining ¼ cup/60 ml of the olive oil into the red onion mixture, season with salt, and divide this mixture among the plates. Top with shelled hemp seeds and serve warm.

185

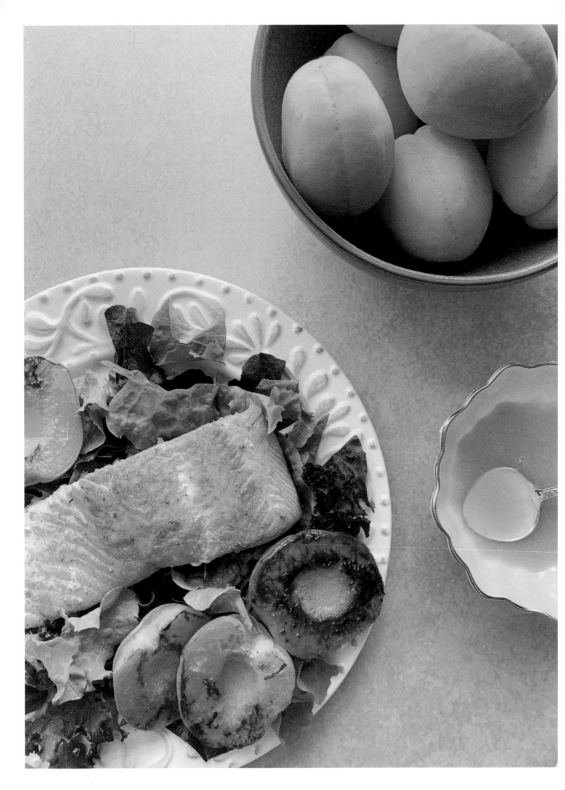

Wild Salmon with Apricots and Honey

Wild salmon is an incredible anti-inflammatory, nutrient-dense food source for your body, beauty, and energy. This delicious recipe takes less than 15 minutes to prepare, start to finish. Briefly cooking the apricots brings out their depth and showcases their sweet-tart flavors—it's worth waiting to find them in season but, if needed, you could substitute other types of stone fruit, such as peaches, nectarines, or plums.

SERVES 2

2 (4-ounce/120 g) skin-on wild salmon fillets

Unrefined salt

1 teaspoon grass-fed organic butter, ghee, or coconut oil

3 tablespoons/scant 50 ml freshly squeezed lemon juice, divided

4 ripe apricots, pitted and halved

1 tablespoon raw honey

1 teaspoon whole-grain mustard

2 large handfuls salad greens

Rinse and dry the salmon and season with the salt. Melt the butter in a large skillet over medium heat. Add the salmon, skin-side down, and let cook, uncovered, until the fillets are almost fully opaque and the skin is crisp, 6 to 8 minutes depending on their thickness. Flip the fillets and cook the top sides for 2 minutes more. Remove the salmon from the pan.

Lower the heat to low, add 1 tablespoon of the lemon juice to deglaze the pan, and immediately add apricots, flat-side down. Cook for about 2 minutes, or until warm and browned on cooked side.

While the salmon and apricots cook, whisk together the honey, remaining 2 tablespoons/scant 40 ml of the lemon juice, and mustard in a bowl and season with salt. To serve, divide the greens between 2 plates and top each with a salmon fillet, 4 apricot halves, and a generous drizzle of the honey mixture.

Toasted Pumpkin Seed Pesto Pasta with Balsamic Mushrooms

This dish is such a crowd-pleaser, with all of the intense basil flavor of traditional pesto, but with the added depth (and mega-nutrition) of freshly toasted pumpkin seeds and handfuls of greens. I love the contrast of nutty, bright pesto and tangy, umami balsamic mushrooms. Make it with chickpea or lentil pasta for tons of additional protein.

SERVES 4

2/3 cup/90 g raw pumpkin seeds/pepitas

½ cup plus 1 tablespoon/140 ml olive oil

2 garlic cloves, chopped, divided

3 large handfuls (about 3 ounces/90 g) fresh spinach (or sub other leafy greens, such as kale, watercress, or arugula)

1 cup packed/30 g fresh basil leaves

¼ cup/20 g nutritional yeast

½ teaspoon unrefined salt

14 ounces/400 g chopped mushrooms (try a mix of shiitake, cremini, and white button)

2 large portobello mushroom caps (about 6 ounce/170 g), sliced

1 tablespoon low-sodium tamari

1 tablespoon balsamic vinegar

9 ounces/250 g uncooked pasta (I recommend chickpea or lentil varieties)

Heat the pumpkin seeds in a large skillet over medium-low heat until they begin to brown lightly. Remove from the heat and cool slightly. In a high-powered blender or food processor, combine ½ cup/70 g of the toasted pumpkin seeds (reserve the rest for topping), ½ cup/120 ml of the olive oil, half of the chopped garlic, and the greens, basil, nutritional yeast, and salt until all have been incorporated. Set aside.

Return the skillet to medium-low heat, add 1 tablespoon of the olive oil, and heat until warm. Add the remain-

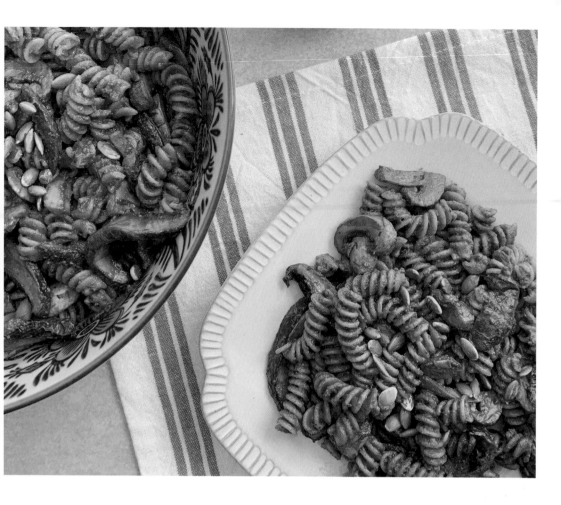

ing chopped garlic and cook until fragrant. Add the chopped mushrooms and stir to coat. Once the mushrooms have warmed, about 3 minutes, pour in the tamari. Cook over medium-low heat until mushrooms have reduced and the liquid has evaporated, about 10 minutes (you can speed the process by pouring off the remaining liquid, if you're short on time). Remove from the heat and pour the balsamic vinegar over the cooked mushrooms, stirring to coat.

Meanwhile, bring a medium pot of salted water to a boil. Add the pasta and cook, stirring occasionally, until it reaches your desired texture. Drain and toss with the pesto and mushrooms. Top with the remaining toasted pumpkin seeds and serve hot.

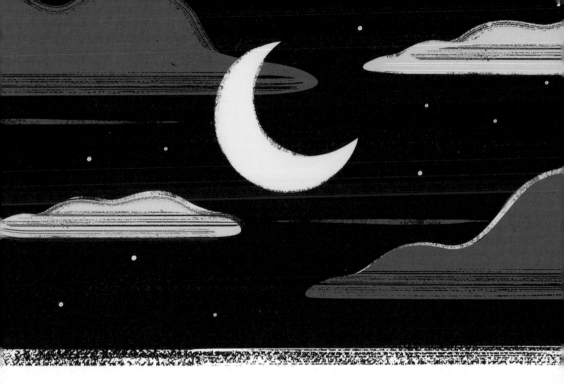

chapter five

Moonlight

In moonlight hours, we turn inward.

Moonlight shines a celestial brilliance over your world. At the same time, darkness sinks in, casting shadows and silvery silhouettes of familiar objects and places and perhaps even bringing feelings of fear and insecurity that threaten your bright energy. Gazing at the moon and stars shining hundreds of thousands of miles away calls to mind our tiny place in a boundless universe. Moonlight reminds us that the same twinkling stars that once guided sailors and explorers still shine and will continue to do so long after our lifetimes. It humbles us into awed silence.

Moonlight also welcomes you with comforting arms. You've spent time on intention and goal-setting, creativity and connection, joy and comfort, and now here is your moment for stillness. For the first time today, the arrival of moonlight grants permission to reflect and to digest the events of the past 16 hours. See whether you can spend some time alone during the moonlight portion of your day to create space for reflection. As you think over the energy of your day, try filling in this statement: Today, I noticed how much my energy is brightened by _____. I also noticed that it's dimmed by _____. When you look back over your day, what do you notice about the energetic highs and lows that you felt? What will you do again tomorrow, and what will you try not to repeat?

When moonlight, or any part of your reflection on your day, yourself, or your life, feels dark, remember to look for and choose light. Although that might mean literally turning on a lamp, it could also mean shifting your thoughts and emotions to a place of joy, wellness, and peace. You are exactly where you are meant to be in this moment. The light is there, even at moments when it seems to be missing. Another sun is already on its way to the horizon.

MOONLIGHT ENERGY THEMES

letting go · releasing · recharging · slowing down · internalizing · digesting · resting · reflecting · repairing · restoring · sleeping

REFLECT ON YOUR MOONLIGHT ENERGY

What ritual(s) do I have to end my day with purpose?

What is my energy like at the close of my day?

Do I snack or eat meals close to bedtime?

What's my sleep environment like?

What's often on my mind as I fall asleep?

How is my overall sleep quality?

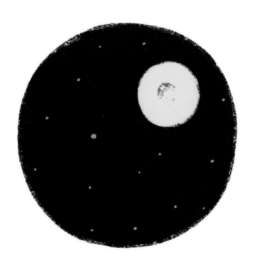

Nature's Energy:
Moon, Stars, and Darkness

Often we turn indoors, draw the curtains, and put up walls to nature when darkness arrives. It's true that the darkest period of our day can be just that—dark, lonely, and fearful—if viewed through the wrong lens. But there's so much magic, and so much light, in stepping outside to experience nature in the moonlight of the day. Tonight, start by finding a dark place to look up at the sky. After a few minutes of darkness, your eyes adjust to lack of light and you notice that the sky becomes a multilayered field of stars, satellites, planets—even shooting stars and constellations. Gazing at the moon and stars fosters an extraordinary connection to the magnificence of the universe.

In my mind, the moon and stars represent infinite possibility, universal connection, and impermanence. To think that we've been able to walk on the moon, orbit the Earth, and map the stars pushes the edges of what I believe is possible in my own life. The idea that, no matter our location on Earth, we're able to gaze at the same moon creates a feeling of connectedness that we know is our energetic reality. And the knowledge that we're merely specks of light in the vast universe brings up feelings of awe that work similar to a spiritual practice.

The arrival of moonlight is a daily reminder that nature works in cycles, large and small. Night settles in to remind us of our need for balance; for every light there is dark, for every period of activity there is rest. These moonlight moments are the most yin of the day. Recall that yin corresponds to such qualities as dark, cool, damp, inward, soft, and feminine. This time of day stands in stark opposition to the daylight you experienced 12 hours earlier. Although not all of nature is resting during the moonlight hours, it's the time when many plants and creatures turn inward. And, of course, darkness in nature is a grand metaphor for cyclical darkness in our human lives. We're reminded that for every dark there is a dawn, and even during a long and difficult night there is promise and possibility of a sunrise.

The stars have a mystical quality that have fascinated humans for centuries. They are symbols of wisdom, beauty, and wonder. Perhaps you connect to the stars through zodiac signs that use the alignment of the stars and planets to forecast the future. Or you might connect to the symbol of a star, one believed to have been created five millennia ago. Incredibly, telescopes show that stars appear to have pointed beams of light similar to the simple five-point drawing of a star that we know so well.

Top Moonlight Energy Drains

❋ **Spending too much time with eyes focused on screens**

❋ **Bright lights, loud noises that excite the nervous system and brain**

❋ **Forgoing a full night of sleep to stay up late**

❋ **Binging on TV or snacks to release built-up stress from the day**

❋ **Worries that interrupt sleep**

MOONLIGHT ENERGY INFLUENCERS

The days can pass by at incredible speeds if you don't slow down to experience them. One sunrise turns to seven, the week begins again, then a month and soon a season depart. Moonlight offers a moment to ground yourself into the present by slowing down enough to savor this day before it closes. Often that means resisting the call of the TVs and tablets and instead going within and getting personal, with a spiritual practice that guides and confers deeper meaning to each 24-hour cycle. In this section, we'll look at the energy of spirituality that could play a number of roles, from complicated to comforting, in the moonlight of your day. And before the day closes, you'll support tomorrow's energy by paring down and releasing whatever weights you've picked up today: dim energy, emotions, worries, to-dos, built-up stress, muscle tension. Ahead, we'll look at the most effective ways to cleanse, clear, and release in the interest of a brighter sunrise tomorrow. And we'll fine-tune the energy of sleep, a respite for the four facets of your energy that helps you fully recharge.

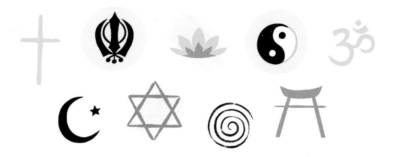

FEEL YOUR PURPOSE:
THE ENERGY OF SPIRITUALITY

What you believe defines your experience of life. Belief not only shapes how you interpret events, it's the lens through which you see your entire world—including yourself. When you look in the mirror and see a divine creation whose existence is a gift intended to bring good to the world, it's harder to single out perceived flaws and shortcomings. **From a spiritual vantage point, the flaws you once identified can be the very gifts that bring you untold joy, insight, and opportunity. Your challenges, your lessons, your dark night could become the ingredients that yield the brightest, most euphoric dawn.** Without the night, the coming sunrise wouldn't look nearly as bright, right? A mindset of possibility founded in your beliefs is an undeniable energetic asset, one that's sometimes the missing link in a journey to feel lit from within.

Creating a spiritual practice of your own enables you to maintain that mindset of possibility along your life's journey. Spirituality expands both possibility and your sense of self. Developing a spiritual practice diverts your focus from the dark, creates deeper meaning in your life, offers guidance along your path, and sets you on track toward the best version of yourself. Your spiritual beliefs may remind you that each moment is a perfect part of your journey, and support you in viewing your life from a place of trust and abundance rather than fear and lack.

What exactly is spirituality, and what defines a spiritual practice? Spirituality itself is a level of awareness, namely, "the quality of being concerned with the human spirit or soul as opposed to material or physical things." It's also your connection to a more conscious existence. Spirituality helps you ignite your light and can even help you sustain it in challenging times. Bringing spirituality into your life actively connects you to your values and purpose, helping you refine your role in life in the process. In so many ways, spirituality eludes definition because it's a deeply personal and individual experience. Rather than direct you to a particular religion (many of which share the same truths) or recommend one form of spiritual practice, I wish to share only the immense value of spirituality in your energetic life. Your spiritual practice may be the most powerful and underutilized energetic influence you possess. Ahead, we'll discuss the foundational ways that your own unique spiritual practice has the potential to light up your energy, and with it, your life.

A Shift in Focus

Nothing keeps you stuck in the dark quite like the inability to shift your focus from troubling circumstances. When you perceive a problem or a hardship, it's often all you can see. Just shouldering the stress, worry, or frustration you feel around the experience is enough to dim your light—and weaken your confidence, your physical body, or your ability to see your way clearly through the situation. That's where a spiritual practice comes in to shift your focus. Grounding your outlook in a belief in a greater plan for your life can balance a hardship with an opportunity or a learning experience, one that allows you a bigger say in your story. Shaking up the comfort of our lives is something that few of us are willing to do unprompted. But given a major challenge or setback, we often rise to the situation and through that experience find ourselves shining brighter than before. Physically, such a shift in perspective prompts the body to lower blood pressure, increase blood flow to the brain for a cognitive boost, and improve immune function to allow healing and thriving to take place.

The next time you're facing a challenge, aim to view it as a learning experience and opportunity. I believe that you're alive to learn, love, and light. Adopting a similar view, in your own way, can help shift your focus from a problem to the possibilities before you. What new opportunities have arisen on this path? Who else can you help along the way? The more you trust in the perfection of this moment, your journey, and what it has to teach you, the more light flows through and from you. That energy can awaken in you almost superhuman resilience, while attracting you to other bright sources of energy along the way.

Perhaps the most fulfilling way to find light in the dark is to bring it to others. It's yet another way to shift your energy, and an act that likely enhances your own spiritual life as a result. Compassion for others has actually been shown in scientific study to be one of the traits most predictive of well-being. Like spirituality itself, no-strings-attached generosity creates a positive energy feedback loop, from yourself to others and back to you. Directing thoughts, resources, and energy toward others has frequently been shown to amplify fulfillment and joy in return. Ask yourself what you have to give without expecting anything in return. It could simply be time or patience. It could be a comforting presence, or appreciation. Often, it lights us up to express the love, kindness, or stewardship that we wish to feel directed toward ourselves as well.

Deeper Meaning

During childhood, there's tremendous focus on the career you'll choose as an adult. What role will you play in our world? As adults, most of us are still somewhere in the process of answering this one. But as you grow, the question that might better serve you is, What's my *purpose*? So many of us fail to distinguish purpose from profession. What if the purpose of our lives is the experience of our journeys? Perhaps the unique experiences and encounters of your life give shape to your purpose. Deepening a spiritual connection encourages you to trust that your life has a purposeful direction, even if you can't define it in the moment. It cultivates strength, faith, and patience while you're in the process.

What does it mean to have a higher purpose? As humans, we inherently seek meaning, explanation, and answers to big questions about our reason for being. I believe that we all have the opportunity to contribute to the positive direction of our world. I take strength in the idea that, at our core, our lives were created with the goals of spreading and embodying love. Spirituality balances the divine purpose of our individual journeys with the humility and lack of ego that we feel in our role as one small piece of the universe.

It's incredibly thrilling to think about the energetic connections we share, our universal oneness. The same energy that we see in a wildflower or the Grand Canyon or the miracle of the ever-cycling seasons is flowing through *us*. Wild, isn't it? Look in the mirror as a reminder that you possess that same energy, in human form. Reflecting on the smallness of yourself creates a feeling of awe that prompts physical change in your body, lowering levels of the inflammatory cytokines that impede healing and even contribute to depression. Feeling awe can also boost your altruistic tendencies, spurring you to act in pure interest of others by diminishing your own central role in the world. What a beautiful way to raise the light within you and spread that light to others in the process.

Guidance and Surrender

The world can feel scary and overwhelming, at the same time that it's joy-filled and miraculous. We try to plan, see, and predict our way down the right paths. But the reality is that we're not all-knowing or all-seeing; we're human. Spirituality releases the need to control and gives us permission to experience life as a personal journey of learning and development. It frees us from the need to shoulder energy-blocking feelings of fear, burden, and worry. Spirituality itself is a balance between taking charge, and letting go. It's a source of both surrender and inspiration that allows us to release the burdens we carry and eliminate the need to know the answer or see the resolution, helping us maintain energy and momentum in the process.

The idea of surrender may appear as if you're giving in, but it's more like an acknowledgment that you're willing to embrace the big picture, rather than getting stuck in the details. Surrender is a demonstration of your faith that good things are yours, and your trust that your journey will take you to them. Letting go of expectations and allowing your life to follow the path that connects you to your light can be scary, but less so when you trust in both your intuition and spiritual guidance. Maybe your current expectations are not serving you; perhaps something even more transformational is in your future. My favorite act of surrender and an intention that the highest good will come from my life's journey is simply saying, "May God's will be done." Such a prayer is a release, a surrender, and an intention all at once. It's an expression of your trust that if you continually seek to brighten your energy and share that energy with the world, you will receive exactly what you need along the way. Because spiritual tools like prayer and meditation have a well-documented positive effect on the body—speeding healing, boosting mental health, and at times even bringing about unexplained recoveries, they're powerful tools for brightening the energy in your life. And they do more than just support the healing or resolution of an issue in question—they remind us of our connectivity and the greater journey we're on. They create a compelling reason that spirituality should be an important part of your energetic life.

Best Version of Self

When each of us strives to our highest good, we brighten the energy of the universe. That highest good, or best self, is reached over time, by consciously crafting the person you want to be. Striving toward that highest self often feels like it has little currency or significance in day-to-day life. But its value becomes clearer over time, in the feedback loop of light that you create in your life. In the interest of energy, try dedicating at least some of your spiritual practice to self-awareness and the ways that you can live to your own highest good. It may even help you to put into words the purpose you see for your life, like this:

Each day on Earth, I'm alive . . .

* **To learn**

* **To love**

* **To spread light**

* **To support others to use their role for these purposes**

When we all create higher aims for ourselves, we shape a more just, peaceful, love-filled existence—and the entire world benefits. Spirituality helps release the dim energy states of fear, jealousy, want, lack, and so on that block us from so much of the good that's possible in our lives. It also encourages you to release past mistakes that continue to dim your light; to eliminate that baggage that's holding you back from becoming the person you aspire to be. There will still be dim energy states, there will still be regrets, but they no longer bring with them failure or shame—only growth and experience. You are perpetually remaking yourself, with your beliefs as the foundation of the you of tomorrow. Every day, every moment, is a chance to start anew, so take this moonlight moment and begin.

As you explore the role of spirituality in your life, pay close attention what resonates with you—and what doesn't. What creates the feeling of bright energy within you? Maybe there's a belief system that you gravitate toward, or a spiritual experience that you've wanted to try. Make this your moment to explore it, knowing that the experience could offer you a huge influx of energy that makes you feel lit from within. Do you have a friend with a spiritual practice? Ask her about it and learn why it's meaningful to her. Spirituality in your own life can involve creating art, spending time in nature, meditating, writing and studying the words of a prayer or religious text, becoming an active part of a religious community, surrendering worries that otherwise rule your mind, or any number of activities. The role of God, or Source, in your practice will be defined by your beliefs. Your spiritual practice will likely evolve through the chapters of your life. If spirituality is uncharted territory for you, I urge you to approach it as a personal exploration that can offer deep meaning for your life. Each day, aim to spend some time on a practice that you create; perhaps you pair a short yoga sequence with reading a favorite spiritual text, or you mix prayer with a few minutes of visualization or quiet breathing.

My biggest spiritual energy shift came when:
I found that surrendering the very real fears around my future with chronic illness was the key to a change in energy and healing capacity.

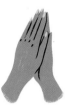

SPIRITUALITY ENERGY IN PRACTICE: GRATITUDE PRAYER

Spirituality takes on a greater role in your life the more you connect to it. It requires attention—a frequent awareness of its presence and function in your life. I think that spirituality feels more natural and fundamental as you integrate it more fully into your day, rather than keeping it separate or compartmentalizing your spiritual self. It helps to have a regular time and place to check in, as with prayer.

Prayer is a universal language. It can be simply "an earnest request or wish," as the Merriam-Webster dictionary defines it. But more often that request is directed specifically toward God, Source, the universe, or a higher power. Science struggles to fully explain the effects of prayer, even as it continues to document its often-profound healing potential. Scientific study has found that even if prayer itself doesn't bring about a resolution to what is being prayed for, the placebo effect it produces may. Prayer appears to create healing power that helps us stay healthier longer, recover faster, and improve our overall quality of life, with particularly strong benefits for mental health and resilience.

Use your moonlight time to create a simple prayer of gratitude for the four facets of your energy. It might go something like this:

Thank you, God, for my physical abilities.
Thank you for the hundreds of strong steps I took today.

Thank you for my mental focus, and for the project
I made great progress on.

*Thank you for the emotions I experience. Thank you in
particular for the joy I felt today in when I visited my nieces.*

*Thank you for the gift of my soul's purpose, and for
the opportunity to continually seek it.*

*Wherever the new day takes me, may my thoughts, actions, and
interactions be in alignment with my higher purpose.*

After you've crafted your prayer, go ahead and say it aloud—a practice that many cultures believe amplifies the experience and its intentions. Feel the surrender and the possibility that comes with it. Gratitude makes you feel alive, vital, loved, flowing with energy. And your personal gratitude prayer can help you feel guided and protected while pushing you to be the best version of yourself and contribute to a better world.

⧽ Energy Booster ⧼

The practice of loving-kindness meditation, also called metta, is one that I love for brightening my energy as I direct good intentions to others. Metta prayer, traditionally a Buddhist practice, is one of the most simple, beautiful, and universal prayer practices, and one you might like to add to your routine.

Metta prayer sounds something like this:

*May all beings be happy and free.
May all beings be well and at peace.
May all beings know love.*

You can pray this prayer, or one like it, by first directing it to yourself "May I be. . .," then to a loved one, a small group, your community, and then to the world.

REBECCA'S MOONLIGHT

NAME: Rebecca Casciano

WHAT TO KNOW ABOUT ME:
I'm a clean beauty makeup artist and founder of the Sacred Beauty Movement. I empower women to embrace their authentic beauty so they can radiate a confidence that positively impacts all aspects of their lives.

THE MOONLIGHT HOURS OF MY DAY ARE USUALLY:
Filled with self-care.

MY ESSENTIALS FOR THE BEST MOONLIGHT ENERGY:
I review my daily wins, big and small, to help me feel more relaxed and positive before bed; I practice a "digital sunset," powering down all electronics at least an hour before bedtime; and my nighttime facial routine is also essential—all of my products are plant-based and they smell and feel amazing!

FAVORITE WAY TO FUEL MY BODY DURING MOONLIGHT HOURS:
Drinking warm lemon water or herbal tea, like chamomile or peppermint.

MOONLIGHT ENERGY INFLUENCERS AFFECT MY PERSONAL ENERGY MOST IN THE AREA OF:
Spirituality. My nightly gratitude practice helps me feel thankful for all of my blessings and connects me to my sacred self, which brings me peace. While I often meditate and pray in the morning, the evenings feel like a good time to reflect and give thanks for another day. This helps me to float into sleep thinking happy thoughts and feeling grounded.

LET IT GO: THE ENERGY OF RELEASE

As you deepen the beauty, resilience, and joy in your life, you'll find that the energy you *let go* is just as important as the energy you take in. Throughout the day, you're continually rebalancing your energy, consciously and sometimes unconsciously, based on the energy around you. And, ideally, you're releasing dim energy or emotions that don't serve you in the process. Still, unwanted energy and emotions get stored and suppressed just as often as they get released. It's not always easy or possible to reflect on the way something is making us feel within the flow of our day, leading us to brush feelings aside. Imagine that your colleague's energy affects you negatively throughout the day, so much so that you don't have much time to separate from it, much less reset your energy. You come home and try to put it out of your mind so you don't bring that dim energy to your relationship, your family, or your home space, but in doing so you suppress this energy even further.

Finally, in the moonlight of your day, you have a chance to release it and reset. If you miss this chance (say, you decide to catch up on emails, do laundry, or watch TV, and forget about it), you'll keep pushing this energy to the periphery, trying not to let it affect you even as it continues to do so. As you close your day, it's so valuable to have at least one healthy practice that allows you to release. And when you let go of unwanted energy, you restore bright energy flow that noticeably lights you up.

Your body's energy, when in balance, flows freely. You default to a feeling of ease. But if you're not actively releasing, it's all too easy to get stuck in a cycle of suppressing and avoiding dim energy until you've built up so much that it takes its toll on one, or all four, of your energy facets. Stuck and suppressed energy manifest in various forms of imbalance—pain, illness, anxiety, restlessness, fear, anger, and sleeplessness, to name a few. Not releasing, forgiving, or allowing yourself to evolve is one of the fastest ways to dim your energy and cloud your joy. Many of us see our past as a major influence, if not *the single biggest influence*, on our present energy. But nothing creates more stuck-ness in our lives today than being trapped by past energy. It's never okay to cheat your-self of today's energetic possibility because of yesterday, making the releasing practices of forgiveness, letting go, and grieving vital to our healthy lives.

FEELING STUCK ENERGY AT THE END OF THE DAY

Unresolved dim energy (think: anxious, angry, overburdened) at the end of the day often leads to dim energy at the start of the *next day*, perpetuating the cycle. How do you know if you're stuck in a dim energy state at the end of the day? You might recognize a pattern like one of these:

Cyclical thinking

Feeling anxious and unsettled

Numbing yourself with food or distractions

Procrastination

Lack of motivation

Feeling unsatisfied

Sadness

Dreading tomorrow

Physical aches and pains

Release is essential for resilience in the face of challenging times. You can't be expected to weather a challenge if you're already carrying around dim energy that taxes your body, mind, emotions, and spirit. Science supports the signif-icance of release, showing that repressing emotions in turn suppresses the immune system, making us vulnerable to a host of health issues. A suppressed immune system diminishes your physical energy in everything from beauty (speeding up the aging process and slowing collagen production that results in visible skin aging) to your body's ability to recover from stress and illness (making you more prone to chronic conditions, mental health issues, and even hormone imbalance that impacts weight, fertility, and mood). Repressing emotions equals suppressing immunity—remember that!

Scientific study shows that our emotions are strong predictors of health outcomes, incredibly even more so than diet and exercise. Emotional traits closely linked to your energy, such as hopefulness, a sense of personal agency, resilience, and taking an active involvement in life, are all positively correlated with health and longevity. On the other hand, systematically avoiding the expression and release of emotions can actually lead them to arise as physical pain or tightness. Somatization is a term used to describe the unconscious process through which emotional pain becomes physical pain, and it can manifest in just about any system of the body. Practice releasing what you'd otherwise hold in. At times when my nervous system issues exhaust me beyond my limits, expressing emotion through movement, journaling, or even tears has allowed me to experience a complete energetic shift. But take note: it's not the *emotions themselves* that threaten to dim your light. Feeling anger, worry, jealousy, and so on is part of the human experience, totally healthy, and makes you no less of a beautiful light shining in the world. Go ahead and feel those emotions; the key is that you experience them when they come to you, acknowledge them, and let them go.

How Can We Release?

Think how amazing it feels to sob at a sad movie, laugh until your abs hurt, punch a pillow when you're mad, sing a song at the top of your lungs in the shower—these are healthy forms of energetic release. Every energy influencer, from spirituality to movement to breath and creativity, includes some component of release. Energetic release takes so many forms—words, actions, visualizations—that you can find one to practice anytime, anyplace. Here's a list of some of my favorites that target each of your four energy facets.

PHYSICAL RELEASE

*Move: run, walk, skip, stretch,
rebound, box, cycle, etc.*

Stretch deeply

Massage—from yourself or someone else

Dance to your favorite song

Sweat in a sauna

Take a salt bath

Practice yoga

Use a foam roller on body muscles

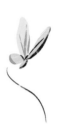

EMOTIONAL RELEASE

Cry it out during a sad movie or song

Chat with a friend

*Watch comedy and laugh until your
stomach hurts*

Yell into a pillow

Forgive

Sing

*Write down your thoughts or emotions on
a paper and then burn it*

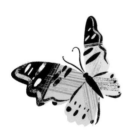

MENTAL RELEASE

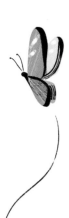

Journal your thoughts

Write tomorrow's to-do list

Prepare for tomorrow morning

Finish a task that's weighing on you

Put down devices

Clean out clutter

SPIRITUAL RELEASE

Pray

Recite a mantra

Paint

Smudge your space

Chant or hum

Spend time in nature

To release most effectively, it's important that you first relax as much as possible. Habits that get you into a relaxed state—think: visualization, meditation, breathing, stretching, singing—are the best friends of release. If you have lots of energy to release, your body might be especially tense, so unclench, unwind, slow your mind, and lengthen your breaths. You might try mentally scanning your body and stretching to loosen up spots where you feel tightness before you begin. As you scan, do you notice any pain or tension? You don't need to spend tons of time evaluating your body, but you may find that it has a default spot for holding energetic tension, such as your jaw, your neck, or your upper back.

Next, practice one of your energy releases. If you're in a place where you can't get up and move around, simply visualize energy moving out of your tense spots and leaving your body. What does it feel like as it leaves? Can you replace the dim energy that's leaving with a bright image or feeling? You don't need to replay every detail of your day to connect this dim energy to its source, simply let it go. Sometimes the release will be brief—a few sentences in a journal or a quick stretch—and other times it will take a while for you to feel your balance return. Spend as long as you like. Easy to moderate exercise before bedtime has been shown to promote deeper sleep, so choose a movement-based release if that's what speaks to you.

Healthy energy release prevents or supersedes other forms of release that sabotage your well-being and happiness over time. Wait, there are *unhealthy* ways to release energy? For sure. You'll recognize them because, while they satisfy you in the moment, they'll leave you with feelings of regret or negativity over time. Think: eating your emotions with junk food or reaching for alcohol before you've dealt with the energy you're feeling. I've found that my clients who can't seem to curb self-destructive nighttime habits—such as binge-eating at night when they're actively trying to lose weight, or staying up too late streaming TV shows that continually lead to disrupted sleep—finally break the cycle when they implement a healthy end-of-day release in its place.

WHO CAN HELP ME WITH ENERGY RELEASE?

If you find that you have much more than just today's energy to release, or if you know that that you have stored energy and emotions from past trauma, you may want support as you explore energy release. If at any point you feel unprepared to deal with the energy and emotions you feel, it's important to seek professional support from a psychotherapist, counselor, coach, or another expert in emotional and energetic processing who can help you safely release feelings that may be especially strong or long-held. In sharing them and letting them go, you're taking important steps to let your light shine as brightly as possible again. If you're looking to explore new or unfamiliar forms of energy release (often called energy work), experts in fields including Reiki, acupuncture, sound healing, and tapping—collectively known as energy workers—can guide you through their own process of energy release.

YOGA FOR RELEASE

Movement can be a very natural way to release, and yoga in particular teaches many poses that encourage energetic release through physical motions and stretches. Try these poses that are especially conducive to energetic release:

Restorative yoga poses, like supported child's pose or goddess pose

Supported back bend

Cat-cow

Thread the needle

Inversion

As you practice release, allow yourself to feel proud and empowered by the choice you're making for your energy, rather than victimized by the unwanted energy that has been burdening you. **See yourself moving through your experience to something meaningful, learned, or beautiful on the other side. Tonight, that is likely a feeling of peace, lightness, sleepiness, well-being, or a restful night ahead.** You might even find that releasing emotions makes you extra tired, making it an ideal bedtime practice.

There are energy releases for all four facets of your energy—physical, emotional, mental, and spiritual—so if you're still feeling tension after jogging around the block (physical energy) or recapping the day over a conversation with your best friend (emotional energy), look at the remaining facets of energy that might need some support. Try jotting down the tasks on your mind to clear your mental energy, or take a few minutes for prayer as a spiritual release. Science has studied several of these forms of release for their benefits to well-being and found interesting explanations for why they work. For example, journaling seems to noticeably engage the vagus nerve and activate the parasympathetic nervous system when practiced for about twenty minutes, three days in a row. Crying it out seems to work because it releases endorphins and oxytocin that can soothe both physical and emotional discomfort and help you sleep better. Choose whatever form of release brings positivity and balance to your body tonight—there's really no single best practice. If it leaves you feeling lit from within, you'll know your body, mind, emotions, and spirit can benefit from release as a regular ritual.

My biggest release energy shift came when:
I stopped returning to work after I put my son to bed, and instead used the time to let my body wind down, release the day, and prepare for a fresh, focused start in the morning.

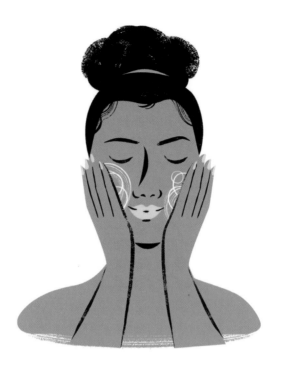

RELEASE ENERGY IN PRACTICE:
CLEANSING SKIN AND BODY

Cleansing your face at night is a habit you've likely been encouraged to practice since your teenage years. On the surface, you're cleansing to remove dirt, sweat, and makeup, and exfoliate old skin cells. But a nighttime cleanse—of your face, or your entire body—is a ritual that takes on larger significance when you couple it with your practice of daily release. The simple act of cleansing stimulates your senses of touch, smell, hearing, and sight; brings fresh circulation to your skin and releases muscle tension; and gives you a symbolic reminder of the release that is so restorative to your energy in the moonlight hours. We all need a regular way to let go of unwanted energy and refresh ourselves, and cleansing is a moment of self-care that achieves both.

My guess is that your cleansing ritual has evolved over time, so let's take that evolution one step further. Why not make your nightly skin cleanse the close of your energetic release ritual? As you cleanse your skin tonight, imagine yourself washing away the unwanted energy of the day, leaving only pure, bright, and light energy behind. Call to mind whatever you're releasing and let it be rinsed or wiped away, refreshing your mind, body, emotions, and spirit. I think that the popularity of the practice of self-care stems in part from our collective need for a regular release ritual. Tonight, create your own self-care practice that embodies this for you.

⋙ Energy Booster ⋘

One of my favorite release rituals is facial massage, especially the practice of facial gua sha. It's ideal coupled with this moonlight cleansing practice. All you'll need is an inexpensive gua sha tool (usually made of polished stone), facial mist, and facial oil. Mist your clean face, press a few drops of oil over your skin with your fingertips, and you'll find that your gua sha stone glides easily, creating an instant feeling of energy release. While you perform this practice, take deep breaths and imagine energy being released with every swipe of the gua sha stone. When you move over areas of tightness, soreness, or tension, visualize the release that's happening in your body to allow energy to once again flow freely. As a bonus, you'll support the flow of lymph (an important waste-removing fluid in your body) and see brighter, smoother, more toned skin. This one works wonders to release my tense brow area, restoring optimal circulation of blood and energy.

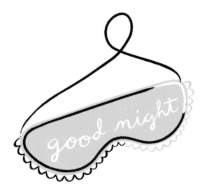

SWEET DREAMS:
THE ENERGY OF SLEEP

Sleep is the bridge between your energetic days; it's the close of one day's energy cycle and preparation for the beginning of another. You know that sleep resets your body and brain and enables you to have the most energetically healthy day possible, but given that personal energy is unseen and unmeasured, it's easy to overlook how dramatically the quality, duration, and frequency of your sleep influence your wakeful energy. Think about the last time you had a restless night. The following day, you probably needed to try so much harder to project bright energy, handle stress, get in the flow of creativity—even choose food with the greatest energy benefits to your physical body. You may have been more rushed and impulsive, less intentional, and maybe you even skipped some of your favorite activities in favor of a nap. **Sleep makes it possible for you to live life as your most beautiful, resilient, joyful self; when it goes awry, bright energy becomes a struggle rather than a flow.**

Sleep is truly one of the most miraculous parts of your energetic day, and certainly one of the top energy influencers to prioritize to perform at your best, recover, and stay well. Yet our endlessly stimulating modern world seems to have been built in opposition to sleep, since we actually need to stop—watching, doing, thinking, working out, planning, shopping, taking in—for about eight hours every night to rest. Insomnia and poor sleep have become an epidemic, and I believe energy has everything to do with the issue. Poor sleep often happens when we have unsettled energy (frenetic, agitated, worried) keeping us from rest. This is one reason that setting a sleep prep alarm 30 minutes *before* bed is so effective. It reminds you to start settling and shifting your energy toward sleep immediately, not 30 minutes later when you want to be dozing off. Your sleep prep can be guided by your specific preferences, but it usually lasts 15 to 30 minutes, involves a calming practice (you can make this one of your energetic releases for the day, such as stretching, journaling, or taking a bath), lowered lights or candles, and peaceful sounds or silence. Rather than missing out on the world, in sleep you're making possible everything your body will experience tomorrow.

It might surprise you that your brain isn't resting at all during sleep; it's actually more active than ever. As your body progresses through sleep stages, your brain is processing and storing memories that contribute to brain growth, as well as cleansing waste, a process managed by the glymphatic system. Without this cleansing process, your brain isn't able to properly detoxify waste that affects learning, memory, and possibly even the future development of Alzheimer's disease. When I'm sleep-deprived, I notice big changes in my nervous system, a key supporter of energetic health. Lack of sleep seriously impacts the nervous system, making you less able to handle stress. Just one night of poor sleep has a negative effect on your brain's ability to regulate your emotional response, making you hypersensitive and potentially far moodier and more anxious than if you'd had adequate rest. In fact, you're seventeen times more likely to have clinical anxiety, and ten times more likely to have clinical depression, if you experience insomnia.

A night of poor sleep also makes you more sensitive to pain, while dulling your body's production of natural opioids that would otherwise lessen your pain perception. The result? You're noticeably achier. You might also get sick more easily, as sleep regulates the immune system. Poor sleep negatively impacts immune system function by depriving us of cytokines that fight inflammation and infection. And on top of that, poor sleep impacts blood sugar and cravings,

increasing insulin resistance and cortisol that makes you crave sugar and processed carbs. The result is often weight gain that could impact your positive
mindset about your appearance and overall health. Each of these is a contribu-
tor to your overall energy.

What if you can't seem to rest well? First, take a look at the stress in your life
and the way you handle it. The body often processes stress as insomnia. It's so
easy to get stuck in a downward spiral: stress begets lack of sleep, which makes
you more prone to stress and continued poor sleep, and so on. But when you
sleep well, you perpetuate a positive cycle: getting restful sleep improves your
mood, which keeps you calmer and makes sleeping well even easier, while good
sleep makes eating healthier and maintaining a healthy weight more effortless.
If you've practiced a healthy form of release from the previous section, you're
already setting yourself up for lower stress and a more energetically restorative
night of sleep. You may also want to add a meditation practice to your day. One
study found that after practicing meditation in the morning, nearly every partic-
ipant fell asleep faster, slept longer, woke up less often, and had more efficient
sleep cycles. Another found 10 minutes of mindfulness exercises to be the brain
equivalent of 44 minutes of extra sleep for those who were sleep-deprived.

Because there are genetic variants that influence our sleep experience, what
helps one person achieve great sleep might be wrong for another. For example,
many sleep experts recommend cooling down your room for your best sleep,
but it's easy for me to get too cool, which keeps me awake in turn. I find it essential to block out all light sources (one of the top sleep interrupters) for my best
sleep, so I keep a soft eye mask in my bedside table and put it on whenever I'm
distracted by outside lights. While light is healing and restoring in many forms,
too much blue light exposure spells trouble for your energy. Blue light that we're
exposed to every time we turn on the television, scroll through our phones,
or read on a laptop or tablet has deleterious effects on the body, suppressing
production of melatonin (the hormone that is important for restorative sleep,
antiaging, and circadian rhythm). Any light in your sleep space disrupts your

circadian clock as well as your melatonin secretion, affecting the length and quality of your hours of rest.

In addition to light, electromagnetic field (EMF) exposure interferes with melatonin production, leading some experts to recommend an EMF-free sleep space. Because EMFs are energetic fields, they have a clear interaction with your own energy. You may find that shutting off your Wi-Fi at night or keeping your sleep space free of devices that emit EMFs allows you more restorative sleep and refreshed energy when you wake. Remember, sleep is your chance to push the reset button on your energy; treat it as the final energy source for your day.

BLUE LIGHT AND BEAUTY

Blue light emitted by phones, tablets, and televisions sets off an inflammatory response in the body and skin that contributes to the breakdown of collagen and elastin (key structural components of skin that give it its youthful appearance and prevent wrinkles), as well as the formation of dark spots called hyperpigmentation. Although blue light in small doses is sometimes used for acne therapy, regular exposure isn't beneficial to our skin. Try switching your screens to a warmer light filter, and make sure your diet contains antioxidant-rich, collagen-building foods, such as leafy greens, pastured eggs, colorful raw peppers, cabbage, berries, or even bone broth. During sleep, the body secretes growth hormones that assist in skin repair and the optimal health of your whole body. When you don't sleep well (because of too much blue light exposure, or otherwise), you miss these youthful benefits.

My biggest sleep energy shift came when:
I replaced nighttime screens with books, magazines, and other wind-down activities

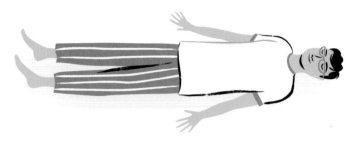

SLEEP ENERGY IN PRACTICE: YOGA NIDRA

Both yoga and meditation offer profound energy benefits for the body, but these practices sometimes feel intimidating to newcomers. One way to gently and easily segue into yoga or meditation is to try a guided relaxation practice called yoga nidra that combines some elements of both meditation and yoga. Yoga nidra allows the body and mind to deeply relax while you remain awake in a deep theta or even deeper delta brain wave state that lets you access your subconscious. The delta brain wave state (often reached in yoga nidra, as well as during some meditation and deep sleep) is one where our bodies release the most antiaging growth hormone, making this practice another fountain of youth. One study used brain scans to show that the brains of yoga nidra practitioners entered a state of profoundly deep relaxation akin to sleep, yet remained awake. Another showed the practice to significantly decrease anxiety and alleviate depression and PTSD. It's believed that 1 hour of yoga nidra is as restorative to the body and nervous system as several hours of sleep, so you could even use this practice during the day when in need of a deep recharge. During yoga nidra, you may experience feelings of overwhelming peace and well-being, which are healing to your body and beneficial to your energy.

Yoga nidra is often practiced in savasana pose, the final resting posture of yoga practice that has you lie on the floor with arms at your sides, palms facing up, and your entire body relaxed. If you prefer, you can also prop yourself up on pillows in a pose that feels relaxed and supported. To explore a nighttime yoga nidra that will begin to relax your body and mind in support of restorative sleep, you only need 10 to 15 minutes. A longer, more restorative practice would be 30 to 60 minutes, and you can readily find guided yoga nidra of that length to listen to at home.

Lie down in a comfortable place, on your back with your arms at your sides and palms up. A soft spot on the floor works, as does a yoga mat or even your bed. If you plan to sleep afterward (or just want to try this practice as a way to drift into sleep), practicing in bed is fine, but know that it may make you more prone to sleep instead of maintaining a state of awake relaxation. You might also want to cover yourself with a blanket, in case your body temperature drops during its stillness.

Once you're comfortable, create a positive intention, known as a sankalpa, for your yoga nidra practice tonight. You'll think about your sankalpa at the beginning and end of your practice, which can help imprint the intention into your subconscious as you enter and exit deep brain wave states of alpha, theta, and delta.

Once you have your sankalpa in mind, feel that thought spread throughout your body. Then, let heaviness take over your body as you connect to the ground or the spot where you lie.

Slowly breathe in and out through your nose. With each long exhale, count backward from 10, all the way to 1. Every time you exhale, let your body sink deeper and feel heavier.

At this point in your yoga nidra practice, progressively relax each area of your body, moving from your head down your body, and from specific body parts to whole regions of the body.

As you move to each new part of your body and relax it, visualize it filling with warm golden light. Let that light bring you peace, joy, healing, or whatever energy you desire.

At this point, you should be feeling deeply relaxed, in a meditative rhythm that requires you only to effortlessly glide your focus from one body part to the next, allowing you to remain in a hypnotic state. Feel any sensations that come up as you scan your body.

You'll finish your practice by gently moving your body out of its resting state, and focusing on your sankalpa one final time as you return to consciousness—or drift to sleep.

The act of increasing attention to both large and small areas of your body, including muscles, nerves, and organs, brings restorative energy to those areas of your body while supporting energy flow and release. Yoga nidra connects you more fully to your physical body even as it relaxes your mind in a hypnotic way. If you enjoy yoga nidra and its benefits and would like to practice it further, I recommend looking for a guided audio practice that you can simply lie back and listen to as you prepare your body for sleep.

⟩ Energy Booster ⟨

Magnesium is my favorite evening relaxation supplement, one that so many of us are deficient in. I get this mineral from food (leafy greens, raw nuts, beans, bananas), supplements, topical oils, as well as Epsom salts. Magnesium relaxes muscles, soothes anxiety, and is essential for the proper function of the hypothalamic-pituitary-adrenal (HPA) axis, which balances your stress response.

More Ways to Feel the Energy of Moonlight

✳ Let the room get dark without turning on any lights.

✳ Sit outside and look at the stars. Lie on your back, adjust your eyes to the light, and appreciate the vastness of it all and the coming period of rest.

✳ Dance, move, stretch to physically release emotion and energy from your day.

✳ Light a candle in a dark space.

✳ Listen to a guided meditation to settle your mind.

RECIPES TO NOURISH YOUR MOONLIGHT ENERGY

The last bites have been taken and tables have often been cleared by this time of the day. In the moonlight hours, the body begins a period devoted to repair and replenishment rather than digestion. If you're feeling well-nourished at this time of day, you won't need more than a little hydration. Still, on occasion, you might find yourself desiring a few sweet bites to end your day, comforting and warming drinks to encourage sleep, or light snacks that will keep overnight hunger at bay and support uninterrupted rest. You'll find those here, along with inspiration for two overnight breakfasts that you can prepare before bed and have ready for your sunrise meal.

> **Ideal foods for moonlight energy:**
> sleep-supporting foods, like tart cherries, nutmeg, chamomile, oats, bananas, walnuts, almonds; calming adaptogens, like reishi, ashwaganda, chamomile, tulsi; "overnight" foods, like oats, chia pudding; and make-ahead smoothies

Dreamy Dandelion Tonic

Dandelion root tea is one of my favorite drinks for a healthy liver—a key organ for detox, skin radiance, and overall wellness. This date-sweetened tonic combines healthy fats for nutrient absorption with protein-rich collagen for youthful skin structure and hydration. Its coziness makes you want to curl up with a mug, which you can do even late at night since it has no caffeine!

SERVES 1

1½ cups/380 ml strong brewed dandelion root tea (I like Traditional Medicinals, or 1 tablespoon Dandy Blend powder)

1 tablespoon almond butter

1 large pitted Medjool date

1 scoop collagen powder

Pinch of unrefined salt (omit if your almond butter contains salt)

Combine all the ingredients in a high-powered blender and process until no date chunks remain. Transfer to a saucepan and warm the tonic to your desired temperature. Pour into a mug and serve.

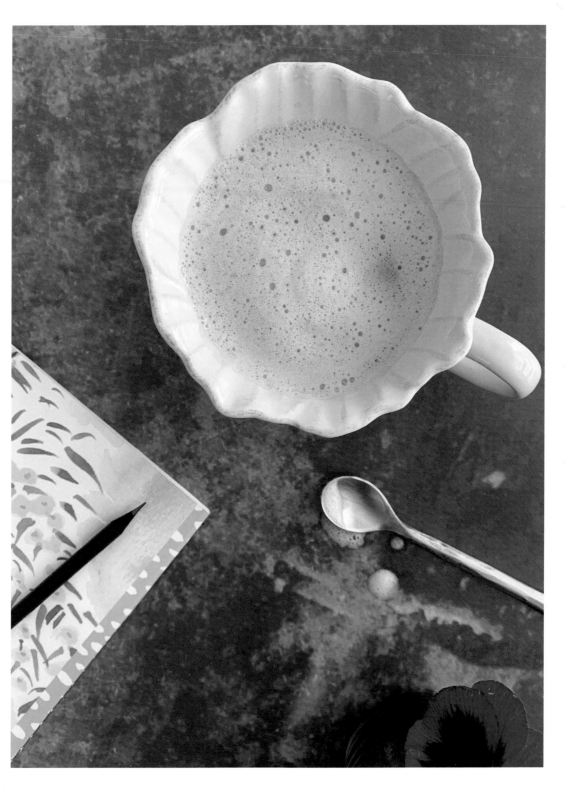

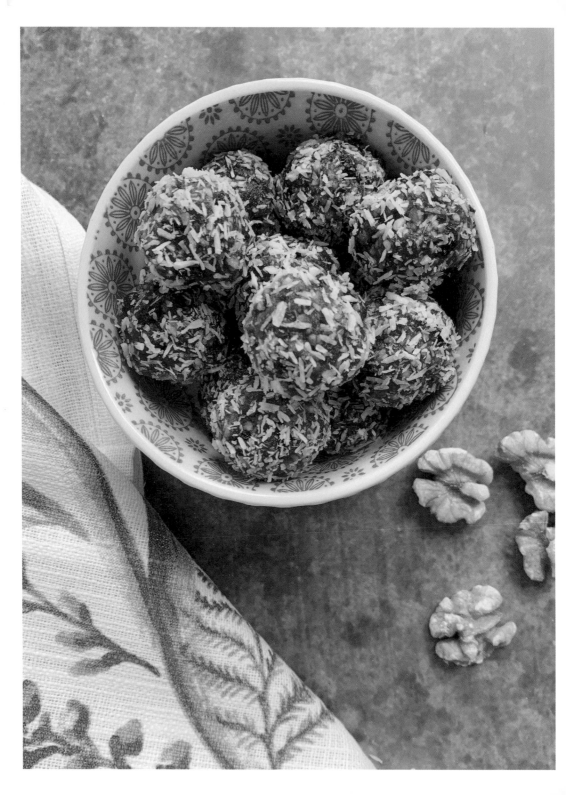

Moonlight Bites

Both tart cherries and walnuts are top food sources of sleep-promoting mela-tonin. Walnuts' rich content of omega-3s may also help keep you full and your blood sugar stable while you sleep. Tart cherries are rich in anthocyanins, which preserve skin elasticity, while reishi mushroom calms your body before sleep.

MAKES 10 BITES

½ cup/60 g dried unsweetened Montmorency cherries

1 cup/100 g raw walnut halves

1½ teaspoons raw honey

½ teaspoon reishi mushroom powder*

Pinch of unrefined salt

Unsweetened shredded coconut, for rolling (optional)

If your cherries are not soft and sticky, soak them for 5 minutes in hot water. Drain them very well, squeezing out any excess water with your hands or a towel before adding them to this recipe. In a food processor, combine the cherries and walnuts and process until the mixture begins to break down. Add the honey, reishi powder, and a pinch of salt, and continue to process, scraping down the sides, for about 30 seconds more. Use your hands to roll the mixture into 1-inch/2.5 cm balls, finishing them by rolling in unsweetened shredded coconut, if desired. Chill and serve. Store in the refrigerator for up to 1 week.

*Omit the reishi if you're pregnant or breastfeeding, and always consult with your doctor before introducing a new functional food into your diet.

Cinnamon Pear Cookies

These cookies are sweetened with pears and dates, giving them more energy and nutrients than counterparts made with processed sugar. Their complex carbs help the body produce serotonin, which supports restful sleep, while cinnamon moderates the blood sugar spike that results from eating sweet foods.

MAKES 15 COOKIES

1 cup/100 g gluten-free rolled oats

½ cup/80 g gluten-free flour blend (I like Bob's Red Mill 1-to-1)

¼ cup/30 g unsweetened shredded coconut flakes

1 teaspoon ground cinnamon

1 teaspoon baking powder

¼ teaspoon unrefined salt

2 large ripe (soft) pears, cored

¼ cup/50 g dates (if not soft, soak in hot water 5 minutes and drain well before using)

½ teaspoon pure vanilla extract

2 tablespoons/20 g dairy-free mini chocolate chips (optional)

Preheat the oven to 350°F/180°C. Line a baking sheet with parchment paper, and set aside.

In a high-powered blender or food processor, briefly pulse the oats to break them apart, then add them to a medium bowl along with the flour, coconut, cinnamon, baking powder, and salt. Stir to combine. Add 1½ pears (set aside the remaining ½ pear) to the blender along with softened dates and vanilla. Blend until smooth, scraping down the sides if needed. Add the purée to the dry ingredients and stir to combine. Peel the remaining ½ pear and finely mince. Add the minced pear and chocolate chips, if using, to the dry ingredients and stir gently to incorporate.

Form the dough into 1½-inch/4 cm balls, place on the prepared baking sheet, and slightly flatten. Bake for about 13 minutes, or until the bottoms turn golden brown. Remove from the oven and allow to cool on a wire rack and serve. The cookies keep in an airtight container at room temperature for 4 days or frozen for 2 months.

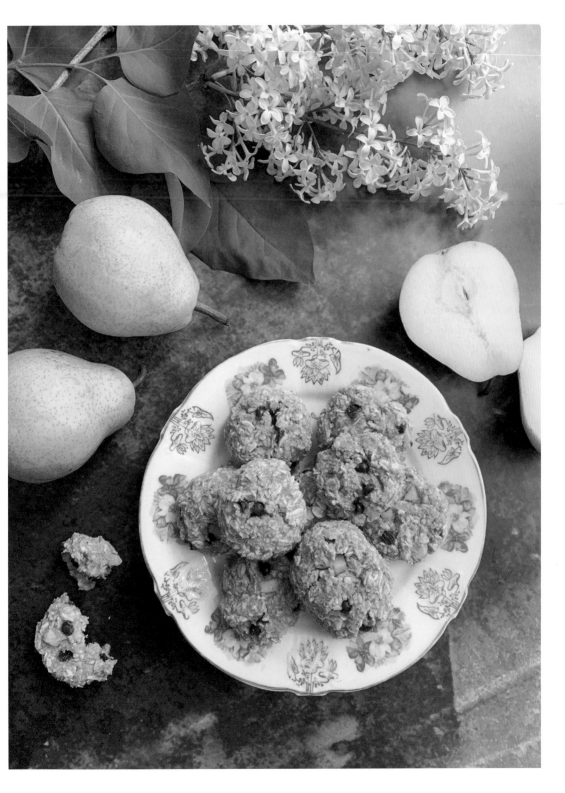

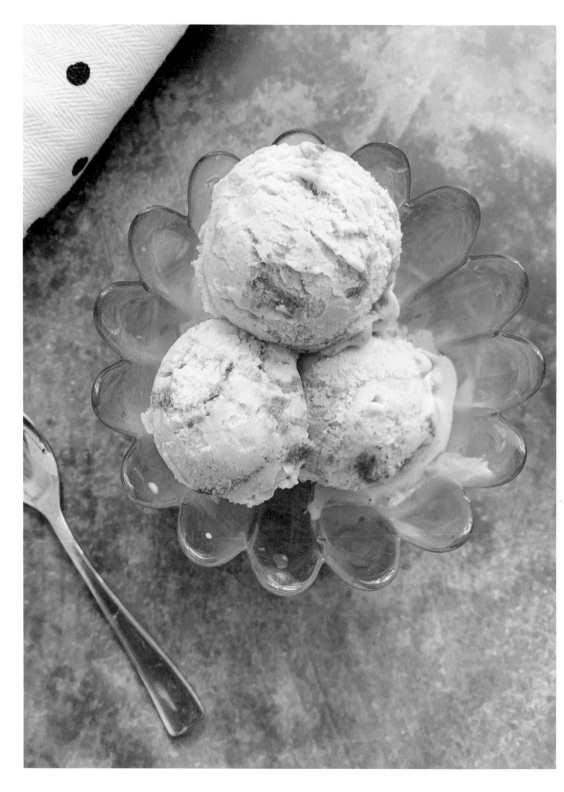

Coco-Banana Ice Cream with Salted Almond Butter Ripple

Bananas make an ideal nighttime snack to support restful sleep and melatonin production. This fruit-sweetened nondairy ice cream gets a tasty twist from salted almond butter that weaves its delicious ripple into every serving. If you feel creative, swap in your favorite ripe fruit (I love it with cherries!) in place of the bananas for endless flavor variations.

SERVES 4 TO 6

1 (13.5-ounce) can full-fat coconut milk

14 ounces/400 g ripe banana, fresh or frozen (about 4)

Unrefined salt

¼ cup/70 g creamy almond butter (add a pinch of salt if yours is unsalted)

In a high-powered blender, combine the coconut milk, bananas, and a pinch of salt until smooth. Transfer to an ice-cream maker and process until frozen to your desired texture, about 15 minutes. Use a butter knife to poke deep channels into the frozen ice cream and pour or spoon in the almond butter until it fills each channel. Turn on the ice-cream maker again for 5 to 10 seconds to swirl the almond butter into the finished ice cream. Serve immediately or transfer to an airtight container and store in the freezer. If frozen for more than a few hours, the ice cream will become solid and require advance time to thaw before serving (allow 10 minutes or more).

Strawberry Super Seed Make-Ahead Breakfast

There's nothing like the convenience of a make-ahead breakfast! This recipe is ideal for fullness, blood sugar balance, and detoxification, not to mention offering an impressive range of minerals that support both beauty and the electrical energy of your body. It takes less than five minutes to assemble at night for an instant breakfast in the morning.

SERVES 1

2 tablespoons/20 g buckwheat groats

1 tablespoon shelled hemp seeds

2 teaspoons chia seeds

1 teaspoon flaxseeds

5 Brazil nuts, roughly chopped

¾ cup/100 g organic strawberries, chopped

1 tablespoon goji berries

Unrefined salt

Pinch of ground cardamom

1 cup/250 ml unsweetened nondairy milk

In a 16-ounce/500 ml lidded glass jar, combine all the ingredients. Close the jar and shake well. Place the jar in the refrigerator to chill for several hours or overnight. Before eating, shake well to evenly distribute the ingredients. Keeps for 3 to 4 days in the refrigerator.

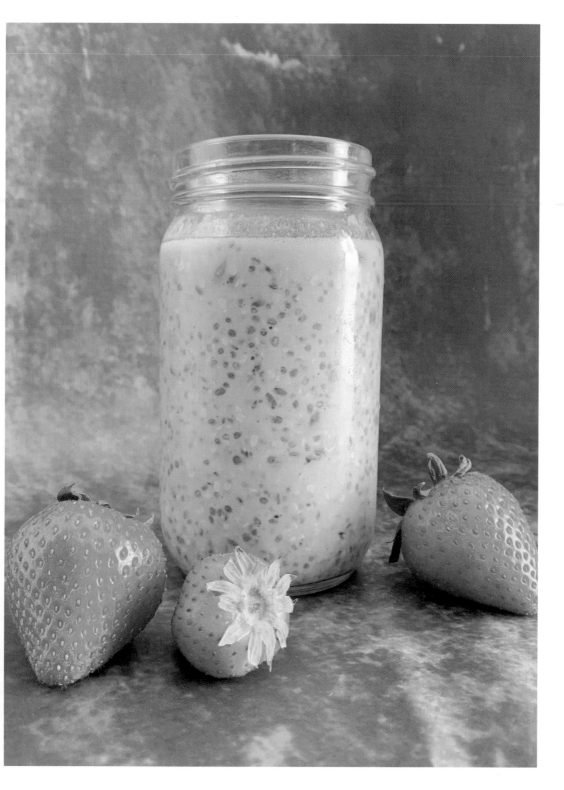

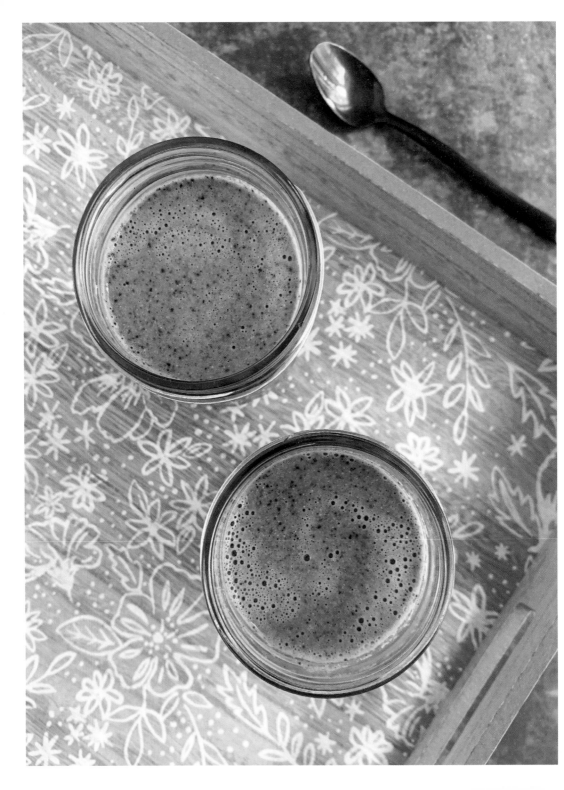

Half Now, Half Later Smoothie

When you hunger for just a little something before bed, make this dual-purpose smoothie, with ingredients that support both restful sleep and an energized morning, then save the other half for your morning wakeup. Ashwaganda in particular improves sleep quality and boosts a.m. brain function, while banana supports both bedtime melatonin production and morning energy. Hemp seeds and sesame tahini are rich in beauty minerals and healthy fats that help you sleep soundly and fuel your morning routine. I like to sip the morning smoothie while I'm preparing a full breakfast or getting ready for the day.

SERVES 1

1 cup/250 ml filtered water

½ cup/70 g frozen blueberries

3 tablespoons/30 g shelled hemp seeds

1 teaspoon sesame tahini

½ ripe banana (about 2.5 ounces/70 g)

¼ teaspoon ashwaganda powder*

In a high-powered blender, combine all the ingredients and blend until smooth. Divide the smoothie between 2 glasses or jars; enjoy 1 now and cover the other and refrigerate overnight for a morning nutrient boost (stir or shake that smoothie portion well before consuming).

*Omit the ashwaganda if you're pregnant, breastfeeding, or have an autoimmune condition, and always consult with your doctor before introducing a new functional food into your diet.

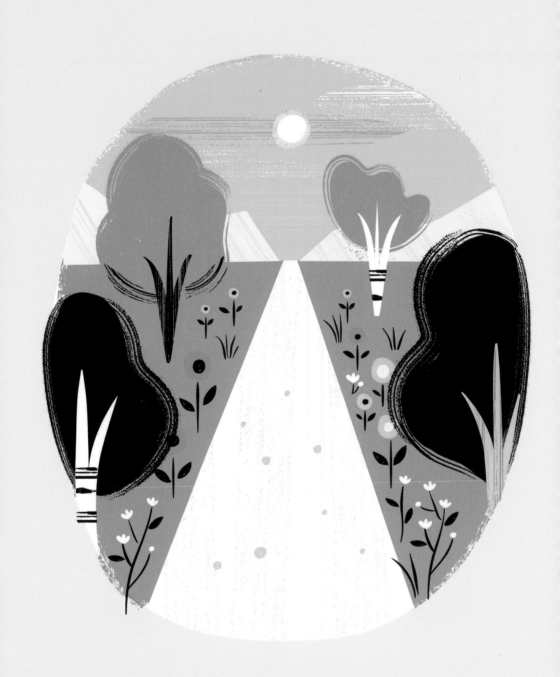

Closing

Life is a string of moments and days, and tomorrow you'll begin again. I'm certain that this book's messages will evolve with you as you journey through your life. One day, it may be a guide to more intentional, joyful living, while another day it may carry you through a difficult time. If you take nothing else from these pages, remember that your light is your power and your choice. It's your guide, it's your hope, it's your strength, it's your glow, it's your spark and spirit. You can choose to flip on its energy sources regardless of circumstance. You have the power to brighten your light with your daily thoughts, actions, and interactions, regardless of whom or what threatens to put it out. Living a life of beauty, resilience, and joy goes far beyond possessions, diets, workouts, and what you see in the mirror. The life you desire is rooted in your energy, and it's free to you and all of us. Unlike the circumstances of your life today, your energy really does define you. Only you have the power to change it every day, in every moment. Make it a healer, a source of joy, a wellspring of beauty, hope, and satisfaction in all that you do. May your light guide you, and others, to the greatest good.

RESOURCES

Connect with Jolene for more recipes and inspiration; for group and individual coaching on nutrition and beauty; and for additional books, classes, and events.

jolenehart.com

Instagram/Twitter: @jolenehart

Facebook.com/beautyiswellness

THE WOMEN PROFILED

Laurel Shaffer: laurelskin.com (page 83)

Nitika Chopra: nitikachopra.com (page 126)

Eminé Rushton: thisconsciouslife.com (page 161)

Rebecca Casciano: rebeccacasciano.com (page 205)

FURTHER READING

Part 1

CHAPTER ONE:
Be the Light You Want to See

p. 23, regarding the heart as a "synchronizing signal": "The energetic heart: Bioelectromagnetic communication within and between people," *Clinical Applications of Bioelectromagnetic Medicine*, 2004.

p. 23, regarding fireflies and resonance: "*Sync*," Steven Strogatz, 2004.

p. 26, regarding anger and its effect on the immune system: "High Immunoglobulin A levels mediate the association between high anger expression and low somatic symptoms in intimate partner violence perpetrators," *Journal of Interpersonal Violence*, February 2016. AND "The role of anger in generalized anxiety disorder," *Cognitive Behavioral Therapy*, March 2012. AND "The physical and mental toll of being angry all the time," *US News & World Report*, October 2017.

p. 27, regarding negativity bias: "Confronting the Negativity Bias," Rick Hanson. AND *"Positivity"*, Barbara Frederickson, 2009. AND "Our brain's negative bias," *Psychology Today*, 2003.

p. 29, regarding the resonance theory of consciousness: "Kicking the psychophysical laws into gear," *Journal of Consciousness Studies*, 2011. AND "The hippies were right: It's all about vibrations man," *Scientific American*, December 2018.

p. 30, regarding universal connection: "The Global Coherence Initiative: Creating a coherent planetary standing wave," *Global Advances in Health Medicine*, March 2012.

p. 36, regarding energy sensitivity: "The highly sensitive brain: An fMRI study of sensory processing sensitivity and response to others' emotions," *Brain and Behavior*, July 2014.

Part 2

INTRODUCTION

p. 52, regarding the effects of beliefs on health benefits: "Mind over milkshakes: Mindsets, not just nutrients, determine ghrelin response," *Health Psychology*, July 2011.

CHAPTER TWO:

Sunrise

p. 58, regarding the UV radiation effects of morning sun: "Morning UV exposure may be less damaging to the skin," *ScienceDaily*, October 2011.

p. 58, regarding the antioxidant levels of melatonin: "Melatonin as an antioxidant: Under promises but over delivers," *Journal of Pineal Research*, October 2016. AND "Antioxidant capacity of the neurohormone melatonin," *Journal of Neural Transmission*, March 2006.

p. 64, regarding the positive emotional effect of smiling: "Voluntary smiling changes regional brain activity," *Psychological Science*, September 1993.

p. 64, regarding the formation of new habits: "How habits are formed: Modeling habit formation in the real world," *European Journal of Social Psychology*, July 2009.

p. 65, regarding the benefits of gratitude: "Strength-based positive interventions: Further evidence for their potential in enhancing well-being and alleviating depression," *Journal of Happiness Studies*, August 2013. AND "Counting blessings versus burdens: An experimental investigation of gratitude and subjective well-being in daily life," *Journal of Personality and Social Psychology*, 2003. AND "Gratitude enhances change in athletes' self-esteem: The moderating role of trust in coach," *Journal of Applied Sport Psychology*, May 2014. AND "Effects of constructive worry, imagery distraction, and gratitude interventions on sleep quality: A pilot trial," *Health and Well-Being*, May 2011. AND "Examining pathways between gratitude and self-rated physical health across adulthood," *Personality and Individual Differences*, January 2013.

AND "A grateful heart is a nonviolent heart: Cross-sectional, experience sampling, longitudinal, and experimental evidence," *Social Psychological and Personality Science*, September 2011.

p. 72, regarding movement and its ability to increase memory processing and storage: "Rapid stimulation of human dentate gyrus function with acute mild exercise," *Proceedings of the National Academy of Sciences*, October 2018.

p. 73, regarding knowledge of the benefits of an activity and its effect on health gains: "*How Healing Works*," Wayne Jonas, 2018.

CHAPTER THREE:
Daylight

p. 102, regarding the benefits of grounding: "The effects of grounding (earthing) on inflammation, the immune response, wound healing, and prevention and treatment of chronic inflammatory and autoimmune diseases," *Journal of Inflammation Research*, March 2015.

p. 103, regarding forest bathing and immune function: "Preventative medical effects of nature therapy," *Japanese Journal of Hygiene*, September 2011.

p. 104, regarding the presence of trees and stress recovery: "A dose-response curve describing the relationship between urban tree cover density and self-reported stress recovery," *Environment and Behavior*, September 2015.

p. 106, regarding creativity, positive emotions, feelings of purpose, and social connection: "Everyday creative activity as a path to flourishing," *Journal of Positive Psychology*, January 2016.

p. 107, regarding the balance of flow state: "The relation of flow-experience and physiological arousal under stress—Can u shape it?" *Journal of Experimental Social Psychology*, July 2014.

p. 108, regarding the entry point to flow: "*Beyond Boredom and Anxiety: Experiencing Flow in Work and Play*," Mihaly Csikszentmihalyi, 1975.

p. 112, regarding reducing exposure to EMFs: "*Zapped*," Ann Louise Gittleman, 2010.

p. 114, regarding mind wandering and unhappiness: "Wandering mind not a happy mind," *The Harvard Gazette*, November 2010.

p. 115, regarding green and creativity: "Fertile green: Green facilitates creative performance," *Personality and Social Psychology Bulletin*, March 2012.

p. 115, regarding nature and creativity: "Creativity in the wild: Improving creative reasoning through immersion in natural settings," *PLOS One*, December 2012.

p. 117, regarding the spread of happiness: "Dynamic spread of happiness in a large social network: Longitudinal analysis over 20 years in the Framingham Heart Study," *BMJ*, December 2008.

p. 120, regarding the physical effects of the presence of another person on the body, and regarding strong friend and family relationships and risk of dying from illness: *"How Healing Works,"* Wayne Jonas, 2018.

p. 120, regarding goal-mirroring: "Goal contagion: Perceiving is pursuing," *Journal of Personality and Social Psychology*, August 2004.

p. 123, regarding the effects of Reiki: "Biofield therapies: helpful or full of hype? A best-evidence synthesis," *International Journal of Behavioral Medicine*, March 2010.

p. 123, regarding the ability of Reiki to activate the parasympathetic nervous system: "Reiki is better than placebo and has broad potential as a complementary health therapy," *Journal of Evidence Based Complementary & Alternative Medicine*, September 2017.

p. 124, regarding the immune benefits of the laying on of hands: *"How Healing Works,"* Wayne Jonas, 2018.

p. 125, regarding distance healing evidence: "Distant Healing," *Subtle Energies Energy Medicine*, 2000.

p. 129, regarding the benefits of vagus nerve stimulation: "Vagus nerve as modulator of the brain-gut axis in psychiatric and inflammatory disorders," *Frontiers in Psychiatry*, March 2018. AND "How positive emotions build physical health: Perceived positive social connections account for the upward spiral between positive emotions and vagal tone," *Psychological Science*, May 2013.

p. 129, regarding the ripple effect of vagal tone: "Paying it forward: Generativity and your vagal tone," *Psychology Today*, June 2017.

p. 130, regarding lack of carbon dioxide: *"The Breathing Book,"* Donna Farhi, 1996.

p. 132, regarding nadi shodhana: "Blood pressure and purdue pegboard scores in individuals with hypertension after alternate nostril breath, breath awareness, and no intervention," *Medical Science Monitor*, January 2013.

CHAPTER FOUR:

Sunset

p. 152, regarding negative ions and seasonal affective disorder: "Treatment of seasonal affective disorder with a high-output negative ionizer," *Journal of Alternative and Complementary Medicine,* January 1995.

p. 152, regarding the effects of positive ions: "The positive health benefits of negative ions," *Nutrition Review*, April 2013.

p. 153, regarding the therapeutic value of flowers: "Effects of flowering and foliage plants in hospital rooms on patients recovering from abdominal surgery," *HortTechnology*, January 2008.

p. 156, regarding playfulness and its link to attractiveness: "A new structural model for the study of adult playfulness: Assessment and exploration of an understudied individual differences variable," *Personality and Individual Differences*, April 2017.

p. 157, regarding humor and inflammation: "Beta-endorphin and HGH increase are associated with both the anticipation and experience of mirthful laughter," *Physiology*, March 2006. AND "Cortisol and catecholamine stress hormone decrease is associated with the behavior of perceptual anticipation of mirthful laughter," *Physiology*, March 2008.

p. 158, regarding the diverse benefits of joy: "Association between perceived happiness levels and peripheral circulating pro-inflammatory cytokine levels in middle-aged adults in Japan," *Neuro Endocrinology Letters*, 2011. AND "A tachykinin-like neuroendocrine signaling axis couples central serotonin action and nutrient sensing with peripheral lipid metabolism." *Nature Communications*, 2017. AND "Positive emotions in early life and longevity: Findings from the nun study," *Journal of Personality and Social Psychology*, 2001. AND "Coping style and depression influence the healing of diabetic foot ulcers: Observational and mechanistic evidence," *Diabetologia*, 2010.

p. 160, regarding acupuncture and depression: "Acupuncture and counselling for depression in primary care: A randomized controlled trial," *Plos One*, September 2013.

p. 160, regarding electroacupuncture and depression: "Effects of electroacupuncture on depression and the production of glial cell line—derived neurotrophic factor compared with fluoxetine: A randomized controlled pilot study," *Journal of Alternative and Complementary Medicine*, September 2013.

p. 168, regarding lemon balm and roman chamomile: "*Emotions & Essential Oils: A Modern Resource for Healing*," 2016.

p. 171, regarding brainwave entrainment: "A comprehensive review of the psychological effects of brainwave entrainment," *Alternative Therapies in Health and Medicine, 2008.*

p. 174, regarding singing bowls before meditation: "Physiological and psychological effects of a Himalayan singing bowl in meditation practice: a quantitative analysis," *American Journal of Health Promotion*, May 2014.

p. 174, regarding Traditional Chinese Medicine five-element music: "Effects of five-element music therapy on elderly people with seasonal affective disorder in a Chinese nursing home," *Journal of Traditional Chinese Medicine, April 2014.* AND "Effects of Chinese medicine five-element music on the quality of life for advanced cancer patients: a randomized controlled trial," *Chinese Journal of Integrative Medicine*, October 2013.

p. 175, regarding brahmari pranayama, humming, and sinus health: "Effects of *Bhramari Pranayama* on health—A systematic review," *Journal of Traditional and Complementary Medicine*, January 2018. AND "Humming greatly increases nasal nitric oxide," *American Journal of Respiratory and Critical Care Medicine*, July 2002. AND "Assessment of nasal and sinus nitric oxide output using single-breath humming exhalations," *European Respiratory Journal*, August 2003.

CHAPTER FIVE:

Moonlight

p. 198, regarding compassion and its link to wellbeing: "Which personality traits are most predictive of wellbeing?" *Scientific American*, January 2017.

p. 199, regarding the benefits of awe: "Positive affect and markers of inflammation: Discrete positive emotions predict lower levels of inflammatory cytokines," *Emotion*, April 2015.

p. 203, regarding the healing powers of prayer: "Prayer, attachment to god, and symptoms of anxiety-related disorders among U.S. adults," *Sociology of Religion*, 2014. AND "Prayers, spiritual support, and positive attitudes in coping with the September 11 national crisis," *Journal of Personality*, 2005. AND "Prayer and healing: A medical and scientific perspective on randomized controlled trials," *Indian Journal of Psychiatry*, October 2009.

p. 207, regarding emotions as strong predictors of health outcomes: "How emotional processes affect physical health and well being," Jefferson Myrna Brind Center of Integrative Medicine.

p. 208, regarding unreleased emotions as physical pain: "Somatization: Diagnosing it sooner through emotion-focused interviewing," *Journal of Family Practice*, March 2005.

p. 211, regarding exercise before bedtime: "Effects of evening exercise on sleep in healthy participants: A systematic review and meta-analysis," *Sports Medicine*, February 2019.

p. 213, regarding journaling and release: "The impact of narrative expressive writing on heart rate, heart rate variability, and blood pressure following marital separation," *Psychosomatic Medicine*, July 2017.

p. 217, regarding the effect of poor sleep on your emotional response: "Chronically anxious? Deep sleep may take the edge off," *Berkeley News*, November 2018.

p. 217, regarding the link between insomnia and anxiety and depression: "The complex relationship between sleep, depression & anxiety," *National Sleep Foundation*, 2019.

p. 218, regarding poor sleep and weight gain: "Short sleep duration is associated with reduced leptin, elevated ghrelin, and increased body mass index," *Plos Medicine*, December 2004.

p. 218, regarding mindfulness and brain benefits similar to sleep: "Close your eyes or open your mind: Effects of sleep and mindfulness exercises on entrepreneurs' exhaustion," *Journal of Business Venturing*, January 2019.

p. 220, regarding yoga nidra brain scans: "A ^{15}O-H$_2$O PET study of meditation and the resting state of normal consciousness," *Human Brain Mapping*, February 1999.

p. 220, regarding yoga nidra and anxiety and PTSD: "Transforming trauma: a qualitative feasibility study of integrative restoration yoga Nidra on combat-related post-traumatic stress disorder," *International Journal of Yoga Therapy*, 2011. AND "Psycho-biological changes with add on yoga nidra in patients with menstrual disorders: A randomized clinical trial," *Journal of Caring Sciences*, March 2016, AND "Delivering integrative restoration-yoga nidra meditation to women with sexual trauma at a veteran's medical center: A pilot study," *International Journal of Yoga Therapy*, 2014.

ACKNOWLEDGMENTS

The journey of this book mirrored my journey of healing in so many ways. It required that so much be let go, that so much be kept in trust, and was filled with dead ends, rock bottoms, and dizzying turns that brought me to an unexpectedly beautiful destination. Thank you to . . .

God, for taking me on a journey of complete transformation you thought I was strong enough to handle. And for reminding me that, with you, I am.

Rob, for never wavering from my side even in those terrifyingly dark years when we had no real understanding of what was happening or how to see our way out. Thank you for always reminding me of my strength, being my lifeline, and holding me through some of the scariest moments imaginable. Every day that I fought for my life, I also fought for our marriage and our future. I love you more than I have words to say.

Jack, for lighting me up with your snuggles and joy, and giving me the chance to be, in your eyes, the most beautiful, fun, and loved mama, even on my sickest days. You have taught me so much about simplicity, joy, and living in the moment. I love you all the way to the universe and God, too. Healing was my only option because of you.

My incredible mother and mother-in-law, without whom there would not be a book, because you helped me balance motherhood and chronic illness and writing when the load was far too heavy for me to shoulder. Watching the love you give as grandmothers reminds me of how lucky Rob and I are to have you as our mothers.

The rest of the Hart, Swanekamp, and Stewart families: thank you for the love and support that lights my life. I am beyond grateful to call you my family.

Readers, the chance to write this book for you has been an incredibly meaningful part of my healing journey, and I'm profoundly grateful to you all for being a part of something so significant in my life. You each have a story to tell and I hope this book strengthens your connection to the wisdom and beauty that lies within you.

My dauntless agent, Clare Pelino, for believing in this project and sticking with it for the two years it took to find the perfect home for me.

Running Press, especially Kristin Kiser, Jennifer Kasius, and Jessica Schmidt, for seeing the beauty in this book, and for welcoming me with open arms by accepting me and my healing journey exactly as we were.

My lovely editor, Cindy Sipala, for helping me shape *Ignite Your Light* into the book it is today. Thank you for manifesting me into your life!

Susan Van Horn and Libby VanderPloeg, for this book's incredibly beautiful design and illustrations. The energy you put into your craft shines through on every page.

Sue Weldon and the staff of Unite for HER, for your endless support, and the incomparable healing community that I'm so proud to be a part of.

The Ladies Floor, for being a place where I could share the ups and downs of my healing journey, and for making Hudson feel even more like home.

Claire Schultz, for spurring me to develop the sun/moon structure of my book proposal.

The many strong, creative women, including Alexis, Katie C, Rebecca, Ali S, Amanda F, Nicolle, and Annie, who lifted me up and cheered me on when things were dark and very lonely. You inspire me.

The many beautiful lights in the green beauty community—too many to list by name—who have offered support over the past few years. I'm honored to know you and I so admire you all.

Those who live with Lyme or invisible illness; I see you and I know how indescribably hard you fight every day. Your strength and grace is incredible. Please keep sharing your stories, and know there are many others out there just like you.

Everyone who has been a part of my treatment and recovery, reached out with words of support, or helped me to keep fighting over the last 10 years. All of you are a part of my story.